KILLING YOU SOFTLY

KILLING YOU SOFTLY

HOW SUGAR IS KILLING US

RICH HOLMAN

RED FALCON
PRESS

Red Falcon Press 2023

an imprint of Red Thread Publishing LLC.

Write to **info@redthreadbooks.com** if you are interested in publishing with Red Thread Publishing. Learn more about publications or foreign rights acquisitions of our catalog of books: www.redthreadbooks.com

Paperback ISBN: 978-1-955683-78-4

Ebook ISBN: 978-1-955683-79-1

Rich Holman

KILLING YOU SOFTLY

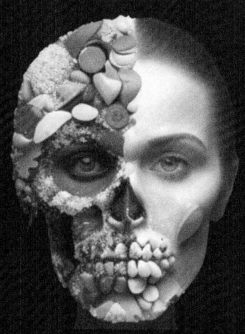

How Sugar is Killing Us

DEDICATION

This book is dedicated to all the people in the world who eat sugar and do not realize how it is destroying their health as well as the health of their families, children, friends, and colleagues. It is especially dedicated to all those unborn babies who are being infused with sugar during their time in the womb and are entering this world with a significant health disadvantage from the time that they take their first breaths.

I have written this book with the purpose of saving at least one life. Hopefully it will be yours.

CONTENTS

PREFACE

SIERRA MELCHER

What if a chance encounter saved your life?
What if a book changed the world?
It is not just hypothetical.

Do you give much credence to chance encounters?

In more ways than one, this book exists as a result of several chance encounters.

One day six years ago Rich was introduced to Dr. Rasa Nikanjam. As a result of that introduction, Rich changed his life, changed his health, saved his life, and was set on a journey of discovery of nutrition, politics, health, and much more. Without that first chance encounter, this book would never have come to pass.

So many people around the globe are suffering from physical ailments, crippled by disease, that we're used to being sick. We're surrounded by sickness and it's become the norm.

The vast majority of the illnesses, diseases, and general sicknesses we suffer with, in the modern age, are preventable. They are not only a result of our diet, they are largely a result of what this book exposes beyond a shadow of a doubt.

Something as fundamental as our health and our ability to live our lives with longevity, and our well-being don't feel like they should be left to chance.

This is your one life. This is your one precious body.

The information in this book is hard-hitting. It's depressing and devastating but it also makes you sit up and pay attention. Thoroughly researched, *Killing You Softly* leaves no stone unturned. Rich Holman passionately shares what he has lived and learned. Shocking and disturbing. There were times I wanted to throw this book across the room.

But. Don't give up!

It is a lot to take in, but there is light at the end of the tunnel, and it is closer than you think.

If you are already convinced or just want a solution to what has plagued you all these years, go to Dr. Rasa Nikanjam's 21-Day Detox Program in Chapter 20. Read all the way through, knowing there is a free practical solution included in these pages. It is not an upsell or gimmick. It is the real deal.

I was already a convert, savvy to the dangers of sugar; diabetes has taken its toll on my family. But I was living in suspended reality and in denial that my daily actions "weren't that bad."

As a result of reading this book, there is no shadow of a doubt that the daily choices I make for myself and for my family are of vital importance. At the time of writing, we are midway through Dr. Rasa Nikanjam's protocol. Only a few days in and I already feel great. She shared it with me herself many years ago but I didn't act on it. Now I am following through on the wisdom available. Not everyone will get a second chance.

If you were given one chance, one opportunity to feel better and live longer; would you take it?

To make better choices for yourself and your family would you want to know? If you had an understanding and the recipe to live a better life, heal, and or prevent so much illness and malaise, would you do it? These are not rhetorical questions.

CHAPTER 1
INTRODUCTION

I have written this book not to make money, not to be famous, and not to change my lifestyle. I am writing to convey a very important truth that 99% of the world needs to clearly hear, understand and believe.

I can already read some of your thoughts, and I bet some of you are thinking how impertinent I am, and who is the 1%? What is the truth that I am suggesting?

For those of you who finish this book, you will truly know that I am not being impertinent, just simply caring. So, you must read on to discover this.

The first question is who is this mystical 1%?

Well, they are those fortunate persons who have discovered that what they put into their mouths each day is critical to their well-being and health and that conventional wisdom is not all it is cracked up to be. This 1% may have had the good fortune to have parents who shared with them the merits of eating real food. Or maybe they lucked out and found an informed doctor, nutritionist, or holistic doctor who set them on the path of healthy eating. These lucky people do not need this book and, in fact, could probably write it. Many may even be working on extending their lives through anti-aging protocols, to be discussed in Chapter 19.

By reading the title of this book and seeing the cover, by scanning the outline, or by reading the dedication, you have probably guessed the truth. Yes, sugar is poison to our bodies and to our health. Sugar kills us slowly, seductively, and softly. It almost killed me conclusively.

I hope at this point I have gotten your interest and attention because I can prove that the perils of sugar consumption are the biggest coverup in human history. But you must read on to understand and to become convinced. I need you to do this for your own health and so that you can share this information with your family, friends, and other contacts.

As I will explain later, your government will not tell you this, and the news media won't tell you. Worst of all, your doctor won't tell you, most likely because he or she may not even know.

If you care about yourself, your family, your kids, your friends and neighbors, you need to know and convey the truth about sugar that has been purposely hidden from you.

Don't give up on me. Read on and be as shocked as I was during my journey in discovering that sugar kills us softly.

CHAPTER 2
BACKGROUND

I am an ordinary person like most of you. I am not famous, not rich, nor am I an influencer. I am not even an author.

I was born on March 10, 1944 which will put me close to, or older than, 80 years of age depending upon when you are reading this book.

I have been residing in Medellin, Colombia since 2007; this is where I wrote *Killing You Softly*, and where I experienced my own personal miracle of avoiding a premature death.

But a little background first. My father was an Air Force pilot, so we traveled a lot. I was born in California and moved shortly thereafter to New York, Colorado, Newfoundland, Virginia, and Texas, where I went to junior high, high school, and the University of Texas.

After graduating from the University of Texas, I served in the Air Force during the Vietnam war and was fortunately stationed at Wright Patterson AFB in Dayton, Ohio. During those four years in Dayton, my fellow officer, Jim Whitten and I, joked about how we had visited many bars, restaurants, and clubs searching for any Viet Cong infiltrators during the evenings, and needless to say, we were successful in preventing any enemy incursions. We were sad that neither of us were recognized with any medals for our extracurricular endeavors. While in the USAF I was able to obtain my MBA from The Ohio State University.

Following Dayton, I spent two years in Boston in automatic test-equipment sales, then eleven years in Atlanta, GA working first as a commodities broker, later as a municipal bond broker, and then as a sales manager for a municipal bond brokerage firm. In late 1983 I married, and we moved to Minneapolis, MN to work with another municipal bond firm. Two years later I was a stockbroker in Los Angeles, and in 1986 I got divorced in Santa Monica, CA. After seven years in Los Angeles, I moved to Atlanta again and joined a former business contact to head up sales for a home repair franchise for two years.

I got my final calling in the United States in 1993 to go to Naples, FL where I literally had three different careers. First, I ran a publishing company where I got to be involved with a lot of public relations and marketing activities, including an appearance on *The Oprah Winfrey Show*. We were able to go public on the NASDAQ and my stock holdings, which were under a sales restriction due to SEC Rule 144, were worth more than $12 million. Unfortunately, after the company's Chapter 11, I ended up with zero for my stock, but it was an interesting ride, to say the least. Next, I did some investment banking and consulting and then, from 2002-2007, mortgage banking.

DISCOVERING MEDELLIN

It was in August 2006 that my life changed dramatically, when I first vacationed to Medellin, Colombia and discovered what I still believe is "the world's best kept secret." It is a city that is one of the nicest cosmopolitan cities in the world, but it suffered, and continues to suffer, from the stigma of the Pablo Escobar days of murder, mayhem, violence, drugs, kidnapping, etc. The success of *Narcos*, on Netflix, as well as some of the international press, continue to perpetuate this stereotype.

I returned in October 2006 and decided that I should buy some real estate before the world discovered what I had discovered and would drive up the prices. I thus Googled "Medellin Real Estate" in English to look for a realtor so I could buy a place while prices were low. Lo and behold there was not one word in English for Medellin real estate, Medellin realtors, Medellin apartments for sale, etc. Nada.

So, at age 63, not being in real estate in the U.S., and not speaking Spanish, I came up with the idea to start a real estate company to serve foreigners. I was originally going to name it First American Realty Colombia until my brother pointed out that the abbreviation would be FARC—not a great marketing moniker. Thus, starting in 2007 with one part-time employee, I launched First American Realty Medellin (FARM).

By 2019 and after several name changes, my company had 110 employees, nine partners, six offices in three countries, and had expanded to include sales, property management, rental building development, agricultural investments, and hotels. Without going into detail, the pandemic and some bad management decisions (not mine, of course) forced a dissolution of the company. As of this writing I am operating a small real estate company (Primavera Realty Medellin), selling Medellin real estate to foreigners, with no employees (six independent sales agents), no office, and no partners, and I could not be happier.

Importantly, something serious happened in 2016. It was something that threatened my happiness and that ended up being the genesis for writing this book.

I discovered that I was dying.

CHAPTER 3
WAS IT LUCK OR WAS IT A MIRACLE?

Hopefully the revelation that I found out I was dying got your attention!

Before I get into that, let's talk about death. I think most of us do not think much about dying when we are young, especially in our teens and twenties as during those times we feel immortal. We think nothing can kill us or that death is a long way away. In our 30s and 40s we occasionally think about it as we notice our waistlines expanding and we have occasional aches, pains, and minor ailments. It is in our 50s and 60s that death seems to rear its ugly head as we start losing some friends and relatives to life's final calling. For those of us who make it into our 70s and 80s, we think about it more and start making plans for this inevitable event.

Personally, I never thought about dying much. I have always been of the younger mindset of living now, enjoying life, and worrying about things later. I have been blessed with great health and had a pretty good exercise regimen in my teens and twenties. I took a break from exercise during my 30s and 40s, and then started weight training after dating a bodybuilder (a woman) when I was 55 years old. We broke up after a short fling, but her legacy was my continuing to lift weights and doing cardio (lots of spinning and step classes). That probably helped save my life, as you will see later.

But at age 72, death came knocking at my door. From my late 60s up to age 72, I saw some disturbing trends, such as my blood pressure increasing; by age 72, it was 160/100. I had lots of aches and pains. My energy was lower. I had a kidney stone attack. One day half my face was numb and I was diagnosed with Bell's palsy. My cholesterol was high. But worst of all were my feet and ankles. Every morning I would wake up and my feet were normal; after an hour or so, they looked like elephant feet. I could barely get my size 13 shoes on. I went to the doctor here in Medellin and he did what the doctors do in the US: he prescribed me pills—primarily blood pressure medication and statins.

My blood pressure medications helped, but overall I just figured out that I was old. Death was awaiting. It was time to prepare for it. I sold half my private stock back to my company to be paid out monthly over five years. My thinking was that this could help me with my medical bills if I lived that long. I was moved out of some key positions in my company (my young partners were sort of putting me out to pasture). I worked at reducing my stress levels. However, every morning I got a big reminder when I looked at my elephant feet that something was wrong with me. I was old, a lot of my friends had already died, and I was probably next.

Living in Medellin, I discovered there were certain items I could not find, like Irish Spring soap, Track Two razors, Noxzema shaving cream, size 13B men's shoes, Dale's BBQ Sauce, books written in English (both fiction and non-fiction), and other items.

I was fortunate to discover that I could buy items online from Amazon and use a re-shipper in Miami to mail these items directly to my doorstep. I love to read. I could survive a desert island or prison if you let me have access to good books of all types. I prefer paper books. I like to turn pages and feel them. After finishing them, I put them in my library and never lend them out unless the person promises to return them and then I only give them one book as they never return the original.

My habit in buying books from Amazon was to check the latest from my favorite authors, then look for books whose names I have written down for some reason, check out some new authors, and review the *New York Times* Best Sellers List (it appears Amazon has now discontinued this). Typically I would buy 80% fiction and 20% non-fiction because.I like to read to relax and not always be working or serious.

Fortunately, in 2016 the *New York Times* Best Sellers List had a particular book that caught my eye. It was a non-fiction book for a category I rarely read, Health and Medical. It was entitled, *Sugar Crush*, written by Dr. Richard Jacoby. What caught my eye was the delicious-looking cupcake with sprinkles with a caption below the cupcake, "How to Reduce Inflammation, Reverse Nerve Damage, and Reclaim Good Health." Of course, the word that caught my eye, with my elephant-sized feet, was *inflammation*.

The name of the book, *Sugar Crush*, did not mean much to me. For 72 years I had been under the impression that sugar was fine to eat. I knew it could affect my appetite as my mom always said to not eat sweets before dinner. Don't we as children get sweets when we are good? To get dessert, we must eat all of our food, correct? In fact, I remember in the mid 1990s going on a no-fat diet to lose weight, which meant I could have my toast with jam on it, but no butter. I did know that sugar causes cavities as I have always had lots of cavities and have put a number of dentists' kids through college with my cavity-driven dental checkups, root canals, and crowns. But I thought sugar gives us energy and a lift. I did not associate it with anything bad other than cavities.

I thought, "What the heck, why not order this book?" as my curiosity was certainly piqued. I remember when the box arrived, I removed all the items and did not open up or even look at *Sugar Crush*. The latest Grisham book caught my eye, and I then moved on to a Nelson DeMille book. Then I talked myself into trying some serious non-fiction reading and opened up *Sugar Crush*.

By the time I got to page 50, I started to realize that sugar may be bad for you. It has 42 different names, and there is a direct linkage to inflammation and diabetes. Dr. Richard Jacoby, a podiatrist and a peripheral nerve specialist, was concerned with how many new cases in which he was having to amputate diabetic feet and why was that on the increase.

But most importantly, I saw for the first time the term *metabolic syndrome*. I now, for the first time, knew what my health condition was called. It was not a "gotcha moment," but simply suggested to me that maybe I need to cut back on sugar. There was no panic. I was not diabetic or even pre-diabetic at the time. Just high blood pressure, elephant feet, low energy, and aches and pains.

Three days later I finished *Sugar Crush*, and this is where the miracle begins.

The day I finished *Sugar Crush*, I took the book to my office and put it on top of my desk. I had never before taken any of my books to my office as I read them at home. I cannot remember why, but I think I had planned to have it handy in my office in case I wanted to discuss it with somebody.

That very first day, *Sugar Crush* was on my desk. I had a 10:00 a.m. appointment to interview a new listing agent named Gus, a bilingual Colombian who had just moved from Barranquilla to Medellin. Before coming into my office, Gus made an unusual request, asking if his wife could sit in during the interview. I found this a bit strange because in all my time interviewing hundreds of people, in the United States or Colombia, I had never had a request for a spouse to sit in. But I said, "OK."

Gus introduced his wife, Rasa, an Iranian who had migrated to Canada where she had met Gus. Rasa was quiet and demure and said nothing during the interview. After the interview I said to Gus that he was hired and then politely turned my attention to Rasa and asked how they met and what her background was. I then found out she was a holistic doctor who had been trained in Canada, Dr. Rasa Nikanjam.

"Wow, what an opportunity," I thought. I realized I had a chance to show off my newfound knowledge that maybe sugar is not so good for us and showed her my copy of *Sugar Crush*. Rasa took one look at the book, another at my slightly inflamed face, and then a longer glance at my elephant feet, and said, "You need to do a detox!"

My immediate question was, "What is a detox?" and Dr. Rasa explained it is a 21-day program where you do not eat sugar or drink alcohol, and you minimize carbohydrate intake. I was doing fine with the no-sugar part as I was never a big candy eater and I knew that I could stop soft drinks, morning pastries, sugar-coated almonds and ice cream for 21 days. Eating low- or no-carb would mean more veggies, eggs, nuts, salads, and chicken and fish, so that was fine.

But no booze! No alcohol, wine or beer...nada. I had to pause and think, "When was the last time I did not have a drink for three weeks or more?" In April 1969, while I was in the Air Force, I had some acid reflux issues and gave up drinking for a month. It had been 47 years. Could I do it again?

Dr. Rasa was kind enough to email me her detox program, and I decided to give it a try. I had no real expectations but thought maybe I would have some improvement in my health, so why not? I quickly determined the program was doable if I could just quit the alcohol. It meant giving up my favorite beverage—red wine—and my occasional beer, margarita, and gin and tonic. One thing that I did like about the program was there was no calorie counting. Eat as much as you like, just no sugar and processed foods, and low carbs.

This is where it gets interesting. The first six days of the detox, I felt weak and lethargic. In fact, twice I left the gym early as I could not complete my weight workouts. I felt a bit light-headed, fatigued, even a little depressed. At the time I did not realize that I was detoxing a poison: sugar. However, I was determined to go the full 21 days.

On day seven the miracle started. I woke up and looked at my feet. They seemed almost normal. For the previous two years they would often look normal after sleeping, but 30 minutes later I looked like Bigfoot. I waited 30 minutes later for the swelling, but nothing happened. An hour later it was still normal. By the end of the day, they were still normal. I could not quite believe it.

The first photo shows my feet for the previous two years.

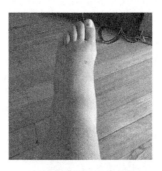

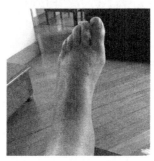

The second photo shows my feet after avoiding sugar and processed food for seven days.

I had this surge of energy. I felt great and went to the gym and, for the first time in a week, I not only completed my workouts but actually added weights to some of my stations. The next day was the same. I was walking faster. My energy seemed boundless. My back pains were gone. Still no swelling in my feet. By day 21, my blood pressure had dropped from 160/100 to 130/80. I felt like a new human being. I weighed myself and had lost 22 pounds all without dieting. I just could not believe it could be that simple. Just quitting sugar. All without dieting!

Was I lucky or was it a miracle? What are the odds of this sequence of events? That I would order *Sugar Crush* because of the picture of a cupcake and the word *inflammation*, have the book sent to Colombia, finally read it, and the day I finish it, interview a new employee while his wife sits in on the interview, find out she is a holistic doctor (I do not recall ever meeting a holistic doctor in 72 years), brag to her about *Sugar Crush* as it was on my desk, she tells me to try a detox, and I was able to quit booze for 21 days while detoxing.

I wanted to know more. Why had this happened? Was I the only one? Why hadn't a doctor told me this? How could I find out more?

I immediately started doing research on the Internet. One thing I am good at is research. It was probably the only real thing that I learned in my MBA program, and it has served me well in life. It quickly became apparent that sugar is not only bad for us, but it is also poison to our systems and builds over time to slowly and softly kill us.

I quickly discovered besides sugar being a poison and a drug, it is the biggest coverup in human history and has killed, and is currently killing, more people over the past 75 years than all the wars, infectious diseases, drug overdoses, drunk drivers, murder, natural disasters, accidents, and terrorism combined. I will show how and why this information has been hidden from us. In the end, there will be no doubt that this sugar travesty, heaped and reaped upon mankind, is really all about the money. Nothing more. Nothing less. Just the almighty dollar. And thus begins my story.

¨DEAD MAN WALKING¨: HOW QUITTING SUGAR SAVED MY LIFE

From 2016 until 2023, those were my years of discovery. I discovered the works of Dr. Robert Lustig, which led me to reading his books and watching many of his videos. I also read books by 23 other doctors, researchers, investigators, and journalists who were basically saying the same thing: that sugar and those products that are laced with sugar, or converted to sugar (like processed foods), are killing us slowly and softly. The more I read, the madder I got. As you will see, we the people do not have informed consent when it comes to what we put into our mouths. We do not know the dangers of sugar consumption.

However, we are led to believe that there are other things more detrimental to our health like eating fat, salt, meat, butter, and eggs. We are told that we should have discipline, count calories, and exercise more—that it is our fault that we are obese. It is suggested that perhaps we need to diet and should try one of the 87 current diets being marketed to us. We hear everything except the fact that sugar and processed foods are not food, and they are bad for our health.

I discovered that for the past 75 years there have been significant lies, subterfuge and misinformation spawned by the money interests of Big Sugar, Big Food, Big Pharma, Big Health, Big Media, and Big Government.

Thus, I have written this book because not only am I mad because the money interests almost killed me prematurely, but because at almost 80 years of age, I am off all meds, in excellent health, my blood work is perfect, and my blood pressure now sits at 120/70. I am living a great life to the tune of, "the last quarter of my life has been my best quarter." It is a miracle I am still alive and I want to give back with this book. If I can save the life of one person, it will be worth it.

Please bear with me as I take you through the facts regarding how we have been lied to, manipulated , and taken advantage of by a heartless system that is destroying our health and lives, all for the sake of profits and money.

I´M MAD AS HELL

You now know the story of how getting off of sugar and processed foods saved my life. I read my first truthful book about the perils of sugar, *Sugar Crush*, by Dr. Richard Jacoby. This was followed by my 21-day detox and the miraculous, almost instantaneous positive changes to my health. I became motivated to learn more.

All the books that I read had the same conclusion: sugar and processed foods are bad for our health and are killing us slowly and softly. I also researched and read more than 500 additionally informative articles, research reports, and podcasts detailing the perils of sugar. These resources explained how Big Sugar has acted much like Big Tobacco, spinning lies and misperceptions. I learned the drastic impact of sugar on healthcare worldwide, how people's lives are being impaired, how sugar is killing more people than all of the wars, infectious diseases, drugs, plagues, terrorism, viruses, drunk drivers, and auto accidents combined. Basically, in their 75 years of mainstream existence, sugar and its unhealthy cousins (high-fructose corn syrup (HFCS) and processed food) are responsible for the biggest coverup in human history.

As I digested all of this information, I had flashbacks to the Oscar-winning movie *Network*, which featured Faye Dunaway and William Holden. The scene that stole the show was when news reporter Peter Finch got up from his newscast, went to the window and opened it, while encouraging his listeners to do the same, and shouted, ¨I am mad as hell and I am not going to take this anymore!¨

Well, that is me. I am mad as hell at the sugar industry. They almost killed me. So, I am shouting to you to get mad as hell and to not let sugar, HFCS, and processed foods destroy your health and the health of your family and friends. If enough of us spread the truth about sugar, hopefully the cacophony of our voices will one day be heard by governments, the news media, and the medical profession.

You may not think there is a sense of urgency, but there is.

A little perspective first. You may not be aware of it, but over the last 10,000,000 years of mankind, there really was very little available sugar other than fructose in fruit and honey. Sugar was cultivated and processed, but it was treated as an exotic spice. It was expensive and not affordable to the masses. You probably remember a lot of old pictures of obese kings, bishops, and members of royal courts who often developed gout and other ailments. They were the only ones who could afford sugar, which at the time was a luxury, hence their inflamed and unhealthy conditions.

The big breakthroughs came when, beginning in the late 18th century, the production of sugar became increasingly mechanized. The steam engine first powered a sugar mill in Jamaica in 1768, and soon after, steam replaced direct firing as the source of process heat.

In 1813 the British chemist Edward Charles Howard invented a method of refining sugar that involved boiling the cane juice not in an open kettle, but in a closed vessel heated by steam and held under partial vacuum. This led to modern industries using multiple-effect evaporators for evaporating water.

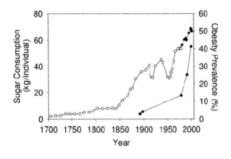

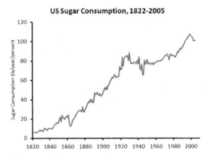

US Sugar Consumption, 1822-2005

Trickle Learning - Nutrition Essentials, US Dept. Commerce &
Labor - USDA Economic Research Service

As you can see in the sugar-consumption charts above, mainstream sugar usage did not really begin until the mid-1800s and did not really accelerate until the early 1920s. This trend was forestalled by sugar rationing in World War I, the Great Depression, and World War II. It was not until the 1940s and 1950s that the processed food industry started to gain a foothold. This was further exacerbated by the introduction of HFCS in the early 1970s.

The period from the 1950s to the 1970s is when we saw the introduction and expansion of such things as TV dinners, fast foods, franchises like McDonalds and Kentucky Fried Chicken; pizza chains; new soft drinks to compete with Coca Cola (e.g., Pepsi Cola, 7 Up, and Dr Pepper); new candy bars like Snickers, Babe Ruth, Butterfinger; and on and on until today, where just ten companies control about 90% of the processed-food business.

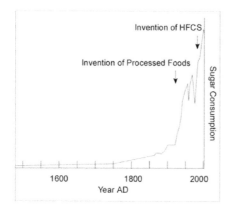

Department of Medicine, McGill University Health Centre

This highly profitable and highly competitive processed-food business has one main tool to hook new customers and get repeat business, and that is to keep adding more and more sugar and/or HFCS to its products.

Now, especially in the United States, we are starting to see the long-term results. In fact, one could say that the United States became the first generation of sugar addicts, beginning in the 1950s after sugar rationing was lifted. U.S. companies began expanding their processed foods and concepts to Europe, Central and South America, and Australia. These populations are now into the second generation of sugar addicts, followed by Asia and Middle East, who are first-genera-tion sugar addicts. In fact, for almost the first time in history we are starting to see obese Asians. Back when I grew up this would have been a rarity.

Now the United States is in its third generation of sugar addicts, and, as will be seen later in this book, the linkage to many diseases is irrefutable. And what are we seeing today in the U.S.? One impact is that babies are being born obese, addicted to sugar, and pre-diabetic. This is despite the pregnant mothers following all the good medical advice: do not smoke, do not drink alcohol, and do not do drugs. So, what do expecting moms do? Eat pizza, soft drinks, ice cream, pastries, and tons of processed foods.

It has just been reported the average life expectancy in the U.S. has been on the decline for five consecutive years beginning in 2017. A baby born in 2017 is expected to live to be 78.6 years old, which is down from 78.7 the year before, according to data from the Centers for Disease Control and Prevention's National Center for Health Statistics. And as of 2023, the US population is down to 76.4 years of life expectancy.

The last three years represent the longest consecutive decline in the American lifespan at birth since the period between 1915 and 1918, which included World War I and the Spanish Flu pandemic, events that killed many millions worldwide.

The pundits blame this on opioids and suicides, when, in fact, sugar is linked to these deaths and many other health-related issues. The key point here is that the long-term damage from sugar is starting to rear its ugly head, and these problems will only accelerate until the world starts treating sugar like tobacco and alcohol. Label it; tax it; keep it out of the reach of children; take it out of the schools, provide public service announcements; educate all pre-school, grade school, high school and university students; and most importantly, provide nutritional training for all doctors and dentists so they can begin to learn how to prescribe real food instead of pills to treat the symptoms of sugar addiction.

The end goal of this book is to convince and motivate you to take action. The proof is in the pudding, and in the case of sugar, it is irrefutable.

CHAPTER 4
WHAT IS SUGAR?

Sugar is a common name for a class of carbohydrates that are sweet-tasting and soluble in water. It is a type of simple carbohydrate and is commonly used as a sweetener in various food and beverages. The scientific name for table sugar, which is the most common form of sugar, is sucrose.

Sucrose is composed of two simpler sugars, glucose and fructose, which are chemically bonded together. Glucose is the primary source of energy for the body, while fructose is naturally found in fruits and some vegetables. When you consume sugar, it is broken down into glucose and fructose during digestion.

We will go into more detail about what happens to your body when you consume sugar in Chapter 9, "Sugar Science for Dummies."

The history of sugar dates back thousands of years.

Ancient Origins: The cultivation of sugarcane originated in New Guinea around 8000 BC. It gradually spread throughout Southeast Asia and reached India around 500 BC. Initially, sugarcane was used for chewing on its sweet stalks or extracting the juice.

Indian Expansion: India became the first center for sugar production and refinement. Indian traders introduced sugar to the Middle East and Persia by the 6th century AD. They developed techniques to crystallize sugar and produce sugar cubes.

Arab Expansion: Arab traders brought sugar to the Mediterranean region, including North Africa and Spain, during the 8th century. They established sugar plantations and mills in these areas, introducing large-scale sugar production.

Crusades and European Introduction: During the Crusades in the 11th and 12th centuries, Europeans encountered sugar in the Middle East. It became a luxury item, and sugar consumption gradually spread among the European aristocracy.

Sugar in the New World: In the 15th century, European explorers, such as Christopher Columbus, introduced sugarcane to the Caribbean and the Americas. The tropical climate was ideal for cultivating sugarcane, and European colonizers established large-scale plantations, primarily using enslaved Africans for labor.

Sugar Boom and Industrialization: From the 16th to the 19th centuries, sugar production grew significantly in the Caribbean, Brazil, and other parts of the Americas. The demand for sugar increased dramatically due to its widespread use as a sweetener and preservative. This led to the rise of the sugar industry, with large plantations, slave labor, and the development of refining techniques.

Sugar Beet and Modern Production: In the 19th century, the discovery of sugar extraction from sugar beets provided an alternative source of sugar. This reduced reliance on sugarcane and led to the establishment of sugar beet industries in Europe and North America.

Industrialization and Mass Consumption: With the advancements of the Industrial Revolution, sugar production became more efficient. It became affordable and widely available, leading to increased consumption and the development of various sugar-based products, such as candies, chocolates, cakes, pies, and soft drinks.

With the advancements of the Industrial Revolution in the 18th and 19th centuries, the manufacturing of sugar underwent significant changes. Water-powered mills and, later, steam-powered machinery were introduced, improving the efficiency and scale of sugar processing. These technological advancements paved the way for large-scale, mechanized sugar production that continues to this day.

The Industrial Revolution began in the latter part of the 18th century and gained momentum into the 19th century; increased efficiency of sugar processing was one of many manufacturing advancements during this time period. This made sugar affordable to the masses and it started seeping into the food supply, especially in the US and Great Britain. WWI and WWII slowed the general consumption of sugar due to sugar rationing during these wars, and there was less usage during the Great Depression.

Anti-sugar author, John Yudkin, best summed it up by saying, "For 2500 years the cost of sugar equaled the cost of caviar, but today sugar costs 1/200th that of caviar."[1]

WHO SPREAD THE SUGAR?

I was born in the United States in 1944. I call that year, near the end of World War II, the beginning of the world's first generation of sugar addicts. This first generation of sugar addicts got to be a part of the 1940s–1960s. This time period witnessed the birth and growth of a number of new industries that started adding sugar to its food, drinks, products, and wares. Some of these categories and companies include:

- **Fast Food** (McDonald's, Burger King, Taco Bell, Kentucky Fried Chicken, Subway, Domino's Pizza, Wendy's, etc.)
- According to Toast, an online news source, there are 194,395 fast food restaurants in the US. It noted that by 2019, 37% of US adults consume fast food every day, 84 million Americans have consumed fast food in the past 24 hours, and one-third of children eat fast food on a daily basis.
- **TV dinners,** also known as frozen meals or frozen dinners, originated in the United States in the mid-20th century.
- The first commercially successful TV dinner was introduced by the American company Swanson in 1953.
- Following Swanson's success, other competitors like Banquet, Morton, and Stouffer's began producing their own versions of TV dinners.
- TV dinners were an instant hit and tapped into the growing popularity of television in American households.

- TV dinners not only revolutionized mealtime convenience but also played a role in shaping American eating habits and the broader frozen food industry. Today, frozen meals continue to be a popular option for busy individuals seeking quick and easy meal solutions.
- **The growth and expansion of processed food companies such as:**
- **Canning Industry:** Companies like Campbell Soup Company and H.J. Heinz Company became successful pioneers in the canned-food industry, offering a variety of processed products.
- **Breakfast Cereals:** Companies such as Kellogg's and General Mills played significant roles in popularizing packaged cereals.
- **Meat Processing:** Companies like Armour and Company, Smithfield Foods, Tyson Foods, Hormel, Cargill, and Oscar Mayer focused on processed meat products such as canned meats, sausages, pork, chicken, bacon, and hot dogs.
- **Baking and Snack Foods:** Companies such as Nestlé, Nabisco, Kraft Food, Mars Inc., General Mills, and Frito-Lay gained prominence in the production of packaged cookies, crackers, dairy products, snacks, condiments breakfast cereals, baking mixes, chips, candy, confectioneries, and snack foods.
- **Soft Drinks:** The soft drink industry experienced significant growth with the rise of companies like Coca-Cola and PepsiCo, who, back in the day, offered 12-oz offerings or smaller, whereas today you can find 32-oz bottles and even 64-oz Big Gulps at your local 7-Eleven.

These are just a few examples of the processed-food companies that were created during the 20th century. The 20th century marked a significant period of growth and innovation, as companies capitalized on advances in food processing, packaging, and marketing to meet the changing demands of the consumer.

The rise of processed-food companies transformed the way people consumed and interacted with food, offering convenient and mass-produced options. However, it should have raised concerns about the nutritional quality and health implications of heavily processed foods. But Big Money shut down this dialogue, and processed food distribution and sales growth continued unabated for the next 75 years.

I was born into America's first generation of sugar addicts. As the fast food, frozen dinner and processed-food businesses (Big Food) started realizing such huge sales and profits, it did not take long to start exporting, selling, distributing, and manufacturing overseas to Europe, Canada, Central and South America, and Australia. Then later to Asia and the Middle East, and even Africa.

It is no coincidence that the United States is now the unhealthiest country in the world despite its great medical advances and spending 4.3 trillion USD annually on health care. The outcomes for America's third generation of sugar addicts are quite disturbing when you consider the following:

- Today's youth in the United States will be the first in the 250-year history of the Republic to not outlive their parents.
- For the year 2021 the United States had total healthcare spending of $3.8 trillion. The next nine countries (China, Japan, Germany, France, United Kingdom, Italy, Brazil, Canada, and Australia) totaled $3.73 trillion.
- Results – Even Cuba is beating us. US life expectancy has fallen to 46th place in the world—below Cuba and French Guiana.[2]
- Many babies today are being born obese, pre-diabetic, and addicted to sugar right out of the womb. This is a direct result of the mother's diet during pregnancy.
- The United States has had five years in a row of declining life expectancy beginning in 2017.
- Despite high US spending, Americans experience worse health outcomes than their peers around the world. For example, life expectancy at birth in the US was 77 years in

2020—three years lower than the Organization for Economic Cooperation and Development (OECD) average. Life expectancy in the US dropped even further in 2021.

- Despite having the most expensive health care system in the world, the United States ranks last overall compared with six other industrialized countries—Australia, Canada, Germany, the Netherlands, New Zealand, and the United Kingdom.
- The United States has 4.2% of the world's population yet has more than 16% of Covid deaths.

However, the rest of the world should not relax as these horrible outcomes are gathering momentum worldwide. For the first time in my life, I am seeing more and more overweight Asians. Diabetes rates are climbing in Asia and the Middle East, especially in China. Forecasts are suggesting more than one billion diabetics worldwide by 2050.

Obesity continues to grow everywhere. For me personally, an interesting side note is what I noticed when I first arrived in Medellin in 2006. The city is known for a lot of things like its year-round spring-like climate, beautiful scenery, friendly people, good infrastructure, excellent health care, low cost of living, and stunningly beautiful women. The Medellin women were not only attractive but were slender in 2006. Their basic diet for the past 500 years in Antioquia, the department or state where Medellin is located, has been the same, consisting of rice, beans, chicken, fish, pork, steak, chicharron, avocados, lettuce/tomato/onion salads, plantains, lots of fruits and vegetables, eggs, coffee, and arepas. A basically healthy diet other than their consumption of breads and pastries in the mornings and occasional soft drinks.

When I arrived in 2006, processed and fast foods were just gaining a foothold in Colombia. McDonald's and Burger King were in Medellin just before me, soon followed by Domino's, KFC, Subway, and other fast-food fare. Soon the supermarket mix changed, with many more processed food offerings and a big expansion of soft drinks, as Coca Cola started grabbing more shelf space. The results are that today, about 50% of the women, and some of the men, in Medellin are now overweight. The trend is getting worse, but in my informal observation this seems to be following the expansion of sugar, fast foods, soft drinks, and processed foods into the Colombian economy. Some have labeled this diet as the Western Diet.

CHAPTER 5
WHO IS THE SUGAR INDUSTRY?

I think it is vitally important to define the Sugar Industry as any entity that profits directly or indirectly from the growing, processing, manufacturing, distribution, sale, or use of sugar. Therefore, I have broken these entities into several classifications as follows:

BIG SUGAR

- White cane sugar processors
- Sugar cane and beet sugar growers
- High fructose corn syrup manufacturers
- Corn growers

BIG FOOD

- The fast-food industry such as McDonalds, pizza chains, and all the chains with processed foods, soft drinks, sugar in their breads, sauces, etc.
- TV dinner & frozen-food industry
- Processed-food industry, which comprises about 70-80% of all foods found in a grocery store or supermarket

- Soft drink industry—Coca Cola is the world's biggest purchaser of sugar
- The powerful lobbyists worldwide who keep the lid on the truth about sugar and control/influence politicians everywhere
- Every mom-and-pop store, stand or street vendor selling sugar-infused products such as soda pop, desserts, ice cream, pastries, bakeries, candy, fruit juices, doughnuts, sugar-laced coffee, etc.

BIG PHARMA

- Pharmaceutical companies who manufacture pills and medicines to treat the symptoms of sugar addiction and chronic disease

BIG HEALTHCARE

- Hospitals
- Doctors and the medical community who are trained to prescribe pills to treat the symptoms rather than the cause
- American Medical Association (AMA), who is greatly influenced by Big Pharma
- American Dental Association (ADA) and dentists who treat patients suffering from sugar addiction rather than the cause
- Health insurance companies
- PBMs (Pharmaceutical Benefit Managers)
- Drug stores

BIG MEDIA

- The news media, who often neglect to report or misrepresent information about the perils of sugar and processed foods as their advertisers/owners are 50-75% from the above list

BIG GOVERNMENT

- Bought-and-paid-for politicians on both sides of the aisle are not doing their jobs like they finally did when it came to Big Tobacco legislation
- Government agencies infiltrated and financed by Big Pharma (Food and Drug Administration - FDA, Centers for Disease Control and Prevention -CDC, National Institute of Health -NIH), Big Food (FDA), and Big Sugar (United States Department of Agriculture - USDA)
- Lobbyists worldwide help keep the lid on the truth about sugar and control/influence politicians everywhere

In this book when I say the *Sugar Industry*, I am referring to Big Sugar, Big Food, Big Pharma, Big Healthcare, Big Media, and Big Government. It is a Big List that could actually be shortened even further by calling it Big Money. But for this book I will call it the Sugar Industry.

LOTS OF BIGS ARE LINED UP AGAINST US

The Sugar Industry makes trillions of dollars per year in revenues and profits peddling a poison that is even more addictive than cocaine. Processed-food products now comprise about 75% of all food products found in grocery stores/supermarkets in most developed countries, especially in the United States. Our traditional sources of reliable health information have been silenced, influenced, or paid off to neglect to provide informed consent about the dangers of sugar and processed-food consumption. The Sugar Industry lobbyists (politicians can´t get re-elected without their money), the complicit news media (whose biggest advertisers are the sugar industry), the medical professionals who receive no nutritional training in their medical school curriculum and are trained to prescribe pills to treat the symptoms of sugar addiction, and world governments, all have failed the public.

The result is the world is being killed slowly and softly while people are suffering and dying without a whimper, not having a clue as to what has caused their chronic diseases.

CHAPTER 6
IT'S A STACKED DECK
THE SUGAR COVERUPS

L et's assume you are a leader in an industry that makes a trillion USD a year in sales and profits and you see a threat to that business. What do you do, especially if your business is a destructive one that negatively impacts human life? Well, that is the quandary of the Sugar Industry—Big Food, Big Sugar, Big Pharma, and Big Healthcare

Thus, the Sugar Industry has misinformed us, lied to us, distracted us, addicted us, and basically done everything to maintain the status quo of creating a sick care system that is highly profitable and one that only makes money if people are sick from eating sugar and processed foods.

Just think about it. The Sugar Industry has a system where a legal drug, *sugar*, which is loved by all and is highly addictive, is put into our food supply system and makes us sick while killing us slowly and softly. Big Food and Big Sugar make money on the front end. Then Big Pharma and Big Health make money on the back end, by treating sick people with chronic disease. What a racket!

In my opinion, the kingpin and, to some degree, mastermind, is Big Pharma. Without their influence, the sick care system would break down. This may seem like a harsh thing to say about an industry that gives the people in the United States their most prized possession—the *pill*!

Yes, the American public, and now other parts of the world, want a pill to cure everything. Yet as Dr. Lustig has pointed out, there is no pill that can do what eating real food can do. One might ask what do these pills do that are so expensively and generously provided by Big Pharma to address our chronic disease healthcare issues? The answer is they treat the symptoms of sugar addiction, not the cause.

The article "How the FDA & Big Pharma Collusion Can Kill Us While Taking Our Money" covers this in some detail. It discusses that Big Pharma is a small group of large international pharmaceutical companies who have taken a large degree of control over what doctors and patients are allowed to use in medical care. Many insightful medical investigations have pointed out these companies have an inherent need to make enormous profits simply to exist. This means that the profit potential of a drug often overshadows the risks and effectiveness of the medication. Overall, this represents a great change in medicine during the past 40 years. The reality is that it is a business and marketing plan, not a diabolical plot. However, it is a business plan using high-octane pharmaceuticals that can kill if not rigorously policed by a third party.[1]

As an organization, the FDA has repeatedly demonstrated an inability to withstand the public and private pressures put on them by the might of Big Pharma. These campaigns for drug approvals are funded by the immense profits Big Pharma reaps through their sales. This issue is compounded and further muddied by the revolving door that regularly swaps personnel between the FDA and pharmaceutical companies that it is supposed to regulate. It really has become like putting the "fox in charge of the hen house."

Since the consumption of sugar and processed foods is destroying our health, wouldn't the simple solution be to simply quit eating these items? The answer is yes, so the next question is, why is this not being done?

WHY DON'T OUR DOCTORS TELL US THE TRUTH ABOUT SUGAR?

In an ideal world we would expect to hear this from our doctors. We would hope and assume that instead of giving us a pill or treatment, they would simply say, "You have to quit eating sugar and processed foods and start exercising." The doctor would ideally be very strict with implicit instructions on how to do this, make the patient accountable, provide a support system, and monitor the progress. But doctors in most cases do not do this. Mine did not when I was dying from metabolic syndrome. The next question is why do they not do this?

Doctors do not do this because they are not trained this way. Fewer than 1% of doctors receive nutritional training in medical school. They do receive lots of training in diagnostic procedures, surgery, and how to prescribe pills to treat symptoms. Not having training in endocrinology and nutrition means they have not connected the dots linking the symptoms of chronic disease to what sugar and processed foods do when they are consumed by their patients. One might now ask as to why doctors do not receive this type of training, and our questionable friend, Big Pharma, rears its ugly head once again.

Yes, pharmaceutical companies do provide financial support to medical schools through various means, and they can have an influence on medical training. Here are some ways in which this occurs.

Pharmaceutical companies fund research projects conducted at medical schools. This funding can support scientific studies, clinical trials, and other research initiatives. While this financial support can be valuable for advancing medical knowledge, it can also create potential conflicts of interest if not carefully managed.

Big Pharma provides educational grants to medical schools. These grants can be used to support academic programs, conferences, workshops, or other educational activities. However, the provision of such grants will come with the expectation of promoting specific drugs or treatments, which can influence the curriculum or the information provided to students.

Pharmaceutical companies will establish relationships with medical school faculty members, such as by sponsoring lectures or providing consulting opportunities. These interactions can create connections between industry and academia, which can influence the educational content and potentially introduce biases.

Big Pharma will offer fellowships or scholarships to medical students or residents, which can provide financial support for their education. While these programs can be beneficial for students, they may also create a relationship between the student and the sponsoring company, potentially influencing their perspectives or choices in the future.

In some cases, pharmaceutical company representatives will serve on advisory boards or committees of medical schools. Their presence can provide insights into industry perspectives but may also influence decision-making processes within the institution.

A not-so-surprising result of a system designed to treat the symptoms of chronic disease rather than the cause is that, in the United States, less than 2% of the 4.3 trillion in health care expenditures is spent on preventative medicine. Just as importantly, fewer than 1% of doctors receive training in nutrition. Perhaps the numbers of doctors trained in nutrition should be 100%? Maybe the percent spent on health care should be 50-75% for preventative medicine?

WHY DOESN'T THE NEWS MEDIA TELL US THE TRUTH ABOUT SUGAR?

The news media today is a diverse and complex ecosystem consisting of various components and in terms of size and influence are ranked as following:

1. **Traditional Print and Broadcast Media:** This includes newspapers, magazines, and major television and radio news networks. This is the number-one source of news for the American public.
2. **Online News Websites:** With the rise of the internet, online news websites such as *The New York Times*, *The Washington Post*, *LA Times*, *Huffington Post*, etc. have become a major component of the news media and have substantial online readerships, offering multimedia content, in-depth reporting, and interactive features.
3. **Cable News Networks** like CNN, Fox News, and MSNBC have significant viewership and are widely recognized as influential news sources. They offer 24-hour coverage of

news events, analysis, and commentary, catering to a range of political perspectives.

4. **Social Media:** Social media platforms like Facebook, Twitter, and YouTube play a significant role in the distribution and consumption of news. Some of these platforms have been involved in censorship activities as noted by the July 5, 2023 ruling by the U.S. District Court for the Western District of Louisiana, granted a temporary injunction barring numerous federal agencies, including the Department of Health and Human Services and the Federal Bureau of Investigation, from contacting social media companies "for the purpose of urging, encouraging, pressuring or inducing in any manner the removal, deletion, suppression or reduction of content containing protected free speech".

5. **News Aggregators:** These platforms collect and curate news articles from various sources, presenting them in a consolidated format. Examples include Google News, Apple News, and Flipboard. Bias and undue influence can exist here as well.

6. **Citizen Journalists** often provide eyewitness accounts, photos, and videos of events as they unfold, contributing to the news coverage and sometimes challenging traditional media narratives. Separating the wheat from the chaff can be a challenge here.

7. **Fact-checking Organizations:** Given the prevalence of misinformation and disinformation, fact-checking organizations have emerged to verify the accuracy of news stories and claims. These organizations can be suspect especially when viewing their cancel-culture efforts during the pandemic in regard to information about vaccines and alternate forms of treatment.

8. **Podcasts and Digital Audio:** Podcasts have gained popularity as a medium for news and storytelling. Many news organizations produce podcasts that cover a wide range of topics, providing an alternative format for news

consumption. There is a growing body of evidence to support the fact that more and more people are using this avenue in the search for fair, balanced, unbiased truthful news.

It's worth noting that these components often overlap and interact with each other. Many traditional media outlets have established a strong online presence and leverage social media platforms for distribution. Furthermore, the lines between professional journalism and user-generated content can blur, raising questions about credibility, accountability, and the need for media literacy in navigating the diverse news media landscape.

WHO ARE THE BIGGEST ADVERTISERS FOR CABLE NEWS NETWORKS AND ONLINE NEWS SERVICES?

Pharmaceutical Companies: Pharmaceutical companies often advertise their prescription medications and over-the-counter products on mainstream and cable news networks. They target viewers who may be interested in health-related news and information.

Consumer Goods and FMCG: Fast-moving consumer goods (FMCG) companies advertise on news sites to promote products such as food, beverages, personal care items, and household goods. Companies like Procter & Gamble, Unilever, Coca-Cola, and Nestle are often seen as major advertisers.

Let's put ourselves into the position of a CEO of a cable news network or online news service when a negative article arises regarding the Sugar Industry, declining life expectancy, chronic disease health care issues, the lack of nutritional training for our doctors, the lies told by Big Food, etc. These stories are either squashed or buried in the health section that is only read by a minority group of healthy people who may read these sections.

Does the old expression, "don't bite the hand that feeds you" come to mind?

WHY DOESN'T OUR GOVERNMENT TELL US THE TRUTH ABOUT SUGAR?

Although this is a growing worldwide problem, I will confine this discussion to the United States as it was basically the biggest initial driver of the Sugar Industry and continues to have the most influence on its sustained growth.

Let´s review first our United States Congress. Our system is set up where congresspersons need to get re-elected every two to six years. To do this they need money, and the Citizens United Supreme Court ruling from 2006 certainly opened up the corporate and lobbying spigot for virtually unlimited funds to be generously provided to senators, congressmen, and congresswomen. For anybody in the Congress to take a stand against the Sugar Industry, it would be political suicide as not only would there be no funding, but also their sugar-addicted constituents would not vote for anybody threatening their comfort foods (sugar, processed foods, soft drinks, and fast foods).

In 2022, the total number of unique, registered lobbyists who have actively lobbied in the United States amounted to 12,644. There are currently 1,834 registered lobbyists working for pharmaceutical and health products, meaning the industry has more than three lobbyists for each member of the Congress and is the largest lobbying group in the US Congress with 15% of all lobbyists representing Big Pharma.

In 2022, the pharmaceuticals and health-products industry in the United States spent the most on lobbying efforts, totaling to about 373.74 million US dollars.[2]

Pharmaceutical and health-product companies poured a record $372 million into lobbying Congress and federal agencies in 2022, outspending every other industry and making up over half of all health-sector lobbying efforts.

About 65% of the Big Pharma lobbyists are former government employees.

Lobbying is also a big business for large food and beverage consumer packaged goods (CPGs).

Coca-Cola, PepsiCo, AB InBev, and 27 other companies spend close to $40 million a year on issues including trade and taxes in an effort to make their voices heard by lawmakers and regulators.

- Total for food and beverage: $27,868,526
- Total number of clients reported: 81
- Total number of lobbyists reported: 324[3]

You can see that Big Food and Big Pharma have a big voice in the US Congress. Thus, we should expect not one little peep from our bought-and-paid-for lawmakers.

THE FOX (BIG PHARMA) IS IN THE HENHOUSE (US GOVERNMENT)

Since we cannot expect to hear anything from our Congress about the perils and poison of the Sugar Industry, how about some voice of reason and concern from our public-health agencies like the NIH (National Institute of Health), the FDA (Food and Drug Administration), and the CDC (Centers for Disease Control and Prevention)?

The United States government has several major health agencies responsible for various aspects of public health, healthcare regulation, and research. Here are some of the key health agencies in the US government.

Centers for Disease Control and Prevention (CDC): The CDC is a national public-health agency under the Department of Health and Human Services (HHS). It focuses on disease prevention, health promotion, and responding to public health emergencies. The CDC conducts research, provides health information and guidance, and collaborates with state and local health departments.

The CDC has accepted millions of dollars through the CDC Foundation, according to the groups behind the petition. During fiscal years 2014 through 2018, the CDC Foundation received $79.6 million from companies like Pfizer, Biogen, and Merck.[4]

Since the CDC Foundation was created, hundreds of corporations have contributed to public-health programs, for a total of $161 million in donations. Many of these contributions could be seen as conflicts of interest—for example, a $193,000 donation from Roche, the maker of antiviral drug Tamiflu, to fund a CDC flu-prevention campaign. The CDC accepted $3.4 million from Pfizer for the prevention of Cryptococcal disease, $1 million from Merck & Co. pharmaceutical company for a program on preventing maternal mortality, and $750,000 from Biogen for a program on screening newborns for spinal muscular atrophy.[5]

Let's say you're a Big Pharma CEO who needs a new leader for your vaccine's unit. Who are you going to call? Gerberding. Yep, Julie Gerberding, former top dog at the CDC. She has plenty of experience overseeing the selection of recommended immunizations. And she steered the CDC ship through more than a few public-health crises. Gerberding, who stepped down from CDC when President Barack Obama came into office, joined Merck as president of its $5 billion vaccine division.[6]

Food and Drug Administration (FDA): The FDA is an agency within the Department of Health and Human Services. It is responsible for ensuring the safety and efficacy of drugs, medical devices, vaccines, biological products, and food and dietary supplements. The FDA regulates and approves these products, monitors their safety, and enforces related regulations.

FDA's Drug Industry Fees Fuel Concerns Over Influence - The pharmaceutical industry finances about 75 percent of the agency's drug division.[7]

Hidden conflicts? Pharma payments to FDA advisers after drug approvals spark ethical concerns. Of 107 physician advisers who voted on the committees *Science* examined, 40 over a nearly four-year period received more than $10,000 in post hoc earnings or research support from the makers of drugs that the panels voted to approve, or from competing firms; 26 of those gained more than $100,000; and six more than $1 million.

Of the more than $24 million in personal payments or research support from industry to the 16 top-earning advisers—who received more than $300,000 each—93% came from the makers of drugs those advisers previously reviewed or from competitors.

FDA has a revolving door: companies often hire agency staffers who manage their successful drug reviews. In a 2016 study in the BMJ (a British medical trade journal), researchers examined the job histories of 55 FDA staff members who had conducted drug reviews over a nine-year period in the hematology oncology field. They found that 15 of the 26 employees who left the agency later worked or consulted for the biopharmaceutical industry. The article that 11 of 16 FDA medical examiners who worked on 28 drug approvals and then left the agency for new jobs are now employed by or consulting for the companies they recently regulated.[8]

Trust issues deepen when yet another FDA commissioner joined the pharmaceutical industry. In June 2019, pharma-giant Pfizer announced that the former US Food and Drug Administration commissioner Scott Gottlieb would be joining its board of directors. The move fell in line with a troubling pattern: after their tenure at the FDA, commissioners tend to go on to advise private companies in the pharmaceutical industry. In fact, nine out of the last ten FDA commissioners—representing nearly four decades of agency leadership—have gone on to work for pharmaceutical companies.[9]

National Institutes of Health (NIH): The NIH is the primary federal agency for biomedical research. It consists of multiple institutes and centers, each focusing on specific areas of health and disease. The NIH conducts and funds medical research, supports research-training programs, and provides grants to academic institutions and scientists.

With an annual budget of more than $37 billion, the National Institutes of Health funds the work of 300,000 scientists across the globe. The NIH receives funding from the US Government and various nonprofit organizations, private foundations, and industry collaborations through grants, contracts, and cooperative agreements. Following are some examples of industry funding to the NIH.

Some pharmaceutical companies collaborate with the NIH on research projects or contribute funding for specific studies and clinical trials. These collaborations may involve joint initiatives, partnerships, or sponsored research agreements.

Biotech companies may engage in collaborations with the NIH, providing funding or resources for research projects that align with their areas of interest.

Companies that manufacture medical devices or develop diagnostic technologies may collaborate with the NIH and provide funding or support for research projects related to their products.

The NIH noted that five more pharmaceutical companies joined the NIH initiative to speed therapeutic discovery. [10]

The NIH Executive Committee is composed of scientific executives representing both US government agencies and industry. It is responsible for overseeing the activities and operations of its four working groups, including reviewing evaluations of experimental agents recommended for preclinical testing and clinical trials by its four working groups and the master protocols designed to test them. Thirty-three percent of the members of the Executive Committee come from Big Pharma.

The National Institutes of Health (NIH) and Foundation for the NIH recently announced they are joining forces with more than a dozen biopharmaceutical companies to boost Covid-19 drug discovery. [11]

Patients who took part in clinical trials at the US National Institutes of Health (NIH) had no idea that scientists at the institutes received $8.9M USD in royalty payments and might benefit financially for the use of their discoveries by pharmaceutical companies and device makers, reports from Associated Press allege. This information was not made public until the press agency obtained the information after filing a request under the Freedom of Information Act.

The press agency has reported that 916 present and former NIH researchers received annual royalty payments averaging $9700 but could receive as much as $150,000 USD. [12]

It is estimated that between fiscal years 2010 and 2020, more than $350 million in royalties were paid by third-parties to the agency and NIH scientists—who are credited as co-inventors.

Agency leadership and top scientists at NIH receive royalty payments. Well-known scientists receiving payments during the period included the following.

Anthony Fauci, director of the National Institute of Allergy and Infectious Diseases (NIAID) and the highest-paid federal bureaucrat, received 23 royalty payments. (Fauci's 2021 taxpayer-funded salary: $456,028)

Francis Collins, NIH director from 2009-2021, received 14 payments. (Collins's 2021 taxpayer-funded salary: $203,500)

Clifford Lane, Fauci's deputy at NIAID, received eight payments. (Lane's 2021 taxpayer-funded salary: $325,287)

Did Collins and Fauci earn these royalties from work performed before their government service or as bench researchers? Are they partial patent owners? If so, what did they contribute to the product's development? If they were rewarded for acting as administrators and not researchers, is it akin to a kickback?[13]

As we can see from the above, there are plenty of inherent conflicts of interest ensconced in the key healthcare agencies within the US Government. Suffice to say it should be pretty clear that the American public cannot expect its government to start warning about the dangers of sugar and processed food any time in the near future. It literally took from the early 1900s to the early 1970s for the US Congress to act against Big Tobacco, and tobacco is so much more obviously harmful than sugar appears to be. But until the American public rises up and demands change, nothing will happen, and sugar will continue to be the slow, silent, soft killer that it is.

The key is informed consent demanding change, and hopefully this book will help contribute to this cause.

CHAPTER 7
HOW THE SUGAR INDUSTRY DISTORTS THE TRUTH

R
emember that the Sugar Industry is anybody who profits from sugar, including Big Pharma, Big Sugar, Big Food, Big Health, Big Media, and Big Government.

There are so many ways that the Sugar Industry distorts the truth that this subject alone could take up an entire book. Distorting the truth can mean a number of tactics like lying, misrepresenting, creating misconceptions, spreading falsehoods, discrediting opponents, distracting attention, bribing, corrupting news and research sources, coverups, etc., all of which the Sugar Industry has done and is currently doing.

Greed, avarice and Big Money often have a co-conspirator: lies. When you look at the "sick care system" in the United States and other countries, you can see the two components of a "sick care" system. The first is a healthcare system that is reactive and not preventative. As discussed previously, doctors are trained to treat the symptoms of sugar addiction, not the cause (sugar).

The second component is the Western diet, which is now prevalent worldwide and which should be termed a "non-food" system. Remember that 75% of the food sold in our supermarkets and grocery stores has sugar in it, quickly converts to sugar, and/or is processed. Food is medicine, and our non-food system is not providing medicine, nutrients, or fiber, but in essence is supplying a substance, sugar, that is destroying our health and lives.

When looking at these two key components of the global "sick care" system we see trillions of US dollars being made in revenues and profits. These are big bucks and, as noted above, when there is Big Money, lies are sure to follow.

These lies can be by design or by omission, and there are many. Are they calculated and by design, or are they from ignorance? From the research that I have personally done, and knowing how money and power corrupt, I believe it is by design. So, let's take a look at some of these lies that have kept the public dumbed down, ignorant, and unmotivated to kick their sugar addictions.

THE WORLD´S MOST BELOVED AND RECOGNIZED TRADEMARK

One of the most beloved brands in the world, Coca Cola, loves to keep not only its formula secret, but also the backstory of how Coke was developed. William Pemberton, the originator of Coca Cola, was a morphine addict as a result of pain treatments from the Civil War. In trying to cure himself he developed Coke with four addictive substances: alcohol, sugar, caffeine, and cocaine (this was after eliminating heroin). In 1903 the federal government eliminated alcohol and cocaine, so only sugar and caffeine remained. After tinkering with salt, caramel, and other ingredients in addition to sugar and caffeine, Coke is now offered and sold in 208 of 209 countries, with only North Korea being Cokeless.[1]

A CALORIE IS A CALORIE

For many years the Sugar Industry communicated through its many publicity outlets that a calorie is a calorie. That it is the quantity, not quality, of calories that counts. The Sugar Research Foundation paid scientists to publish papers exonerating sugar and blaming fat for heart disease. They funded studies showing sugared beverages have no effect on weight gain, whereas independent studies showed just the opposite.[2] Since my undergraduate work was chemical engineering and business, this made sense. It seems to logically follow the first law of thermodynamics—that is, until Dr. Lustig and many other scientists and endocrinologists blew the lid off of this whopper.[3]

FAT IS BAD FOR YOU AND LEADS TO CORONARY DISEASE AND HEART ATTACKS

This may have been the biggest and most destructive lie of all of them, and even today a majority of people think fat is bad for you and causes you to be fat. Makes sense, right? Eat fat and get fat. I am sure that the Sugar Industry loves that the word *fat* serves as both a noun and an adjective. This serves to both confuse and propagate this great lie.[4]

Let's explore a primary tactic of the Sugar Industry: claiming that fat is bad for you, it causes heart attacks, and it makes you fat. This is the tactic that first came to light in the early 1960s and was spear-headed by Ancel Keys, an American physiologist and nutritionist who lived from 1904 to 2004. In fact, Keys's work was embraced by the Eisenhower administration, and a program was employed for President Eisenhower to avoid fats and not worry about carbs and sugar. He suffered two heart attacks during his two terms and a third one after. The no-fat diet did not seem to help the president in that regard; even worse is how the idea that fat is the leading problem for coronary disease became the prevailing wisdom for the next 40-50 years and lingers on even today.

There are seven kinds of fat—some good (omega-3 fatty acids, e.g.), some neutral (saturated fats, e.g.), and some bad (trans fats and omega-6 fats, e.g.).[5] But the bottom line is you need good fat in your diet. You can metabolize fat without triggering an insulin response, and it is not fat that is causing obesity and heart attacks. Just look at the indigenous tribes in the Arctic areas whose primary diets are fat and blubber. They have some of the lowest incidence of heart attacks in the world, and fat is the main staple of their diets.

When studies published in the late 1940s found correlations between high-fat diets and high levels of cholesterol, experts reasoned that if you reduced the amount of total fats in your diet, your risk for heart disease would go down. By the 1980s, doctors, federal health experts, the food industry, and the news media were reporting that a low-fat diet could benefit everyone, even though there was no solid evidence that doing so would prevent issues like heart disease or obesity.

While certain types of fats, including saturated and trans fats, can increase your risk for conditions like heart disease or stroke, healthy fats—like monounsaturated fats (found in olive and other plant oils, avocados, and certain nuts and seeds) and polyunsaturated fats (found in sunflower and other plant oils, walnuts, fish and flaxseeds)—actually help reduce your risk. Good fats are also important for supplying energy, producing important hormones, supporting cell function, and aiding in the absorption of some nutrients.

BAD GOVERNMENT INFORMATION AND MISINFORMATION

- **GRAS (Generally Recognized as Safe):** This is a classification of foods created by the FDA that includes sugar and caffeine and means the processed-food industry can use any amount it wishes with no repercussions.[6] Walter H. Glinsmann, an FDA food scientist, led the approval of sugar under GRAS yet now sits on board of directors of the Corn Refiners Association. He noted fructose as a valuable traditional source of food energy when American sugar consumption in the 1980s was 40 lbs per year; we are now at over 130 lbs per year.[7]
- **The USDA Food Pyramid** (which was changed to My Plate in 2011): For 50 years the USDA put the stuff that destroys our health at the bottom of the Pyramid (grains, flour, cereals, bread, rice, pasta) and the stuff that we can eat and metabolize (butter, eggs, and red meat, e.g.) at the top. Was this perhaps the unhealthiest eating regimen ever developed by mankind?
- **SNAP (Supplemental Nutrition Assistance Program**, aka food stamps): This $75 billion program covers 15% of American adults and 33% of children. Sugared beverages are number two in usage, while numbers 4, 5, 10, 11, and 12 are all foods that contain sugar. As a group sugar-laced items

equal 27% of all SNAP expenditures. People (mostly lower socioeconomic status) using food stamps are 50% more likely to die of heart disease or diabetes than non-SNAP people.[8]
23 Since the vast majority of poor people do not know this, is this a lie of omission?

- Dietary guidelines are still broken and the Government has failed to fix them.

A shocking 48% of US adults are now estimated to be prediabetic or diabetic, and the prevalence of obesity grew from 31% in 2000 to 42% in 2018. How did Americans become such an obese and disease-ridden people in the first place? Increasingly, researchers and even consumers are realizing that it's all about the "standard American (Western) diet," devoid of healthy fats and nutrition, replete with refined grains, ultra processed foods, sugary foods, and drinks. The blame for this belongs with the government, which, beginning in the late 1970s, began to propound the myth that low-fat eating was healthier—an idea that has never been borne out by scientific studies.[9]

SUGAR GIVES YOU ENERGY

Sugar has glucose and fructose. Fructose reduces energy. There are better and healthier sources of glucose than sugar.

SUGARY PRODUCTS ARE COMFORT FOODS

The public has been trained to think of sugary products as "comfort foods." If the Sugar Industry were being truthful, they would change the moniker to, "sugar is a distress food"—the opposite of comfort.

GENETICS ARE THE CAUSE OF OBESITY

Blame it on your parents and not your diet. This is a great deflection by the Sugar Industry.

SALT IS THE MAIN CAUSE OF HYPERTENSION

This misconception distracts from the real culprit, sugar. If your kidneys are working fine, salt will not be an issue as your kidneys will flush out excess salt. But if your kidneys are not working properly, then you will have a problem that can lead to hypertension. What stresses or inhibits your kidney functions? Sugar, of course.

One caveat that needs to be understood is that eating salty items with sugar and high-carbohydrate foods can be extra concerning as salt activates an enzyme that can cause the production of fructose internally. That, in turn, can exacerbate hypertension. Salt in moderation is always a good idea, but sugar is the real villain.

THE MANY NAMES OF SUGAR

I have heard people say, "Oh, this sugar is OK as it is natural." Unfortunately, the truth is that most sugars still basically break down into glucose and fructose, while some others—like lactose and maltose—can still contribute to insulin spikes. In any case, we need to keep our eye on the ball when reading labels to see if sugar is listed as an ingredient.

That sounds simple enough, but your health care provider or dentist probably did not mention there are 56 names for sugar, including the following: sugar (granulated or table), dextrose, fructose, galactose, glucose, lactose, maltose, sucrose, beet sugar, brown sugar, cane juice crystals, cane sugar, castor sugar, coconut sugar, powdered sugar, corn syrup solids, crystalline fructose, date sugar, demerara sugar, dextrin, diastatic malt, ethyl maltol, Florida crystals, golden sugar, glucose syrup solids, grape sugar, icing sugar, maltodextrin, muscovado, panela, raw sugar, sucanat, turbinado sugar, yellow sugar, agave nectar/syrup, barley malt, blackstrap molasses, brown rice syrup, buttered sugar/buttercream, caramel, carob syrup, corn syrup, evaporated cane juice, fruit juice, fruit juice concentrate, golden syrup, high-fructose corn syrup (HFCS), honey, invert sugar, malt syrup, maple syrup, molasses, rice syrup refiner's syrup, sorghum syrup, and treacle. Other than honey, I would be concerned to see any of these ingredients listed on a label of anything I was thinking about eating since none of these sugars feed the gut or protect the liver.

When reading those labels on packaged products, assuming you can read them or that you bring along a magnifying glass, ingredients are listed in order of the highest percentages first. So, if sugar is in the top four or five ingredients, then we definitely should avoid the product. But what if they have three different sugar names lower on the list? If you add them up, they make it to the top three to five positions. Put the package back on the shelf. Now perhaps you are starting to see some of the devious ways the Sugar Industry likes to keep us confused and in the dark: using text for ingredients that is so small you cannot read it, and names for sugar that you have no clue about. These devious tricks are not by accident.

Since fewer than 1% of doctors are trained in nutrition, they do not zero in on the perils of consuming sugar. If your doctor does not know the truth about sugar, how are you supposed to know?[10]

FALSE FLAGS

CCF (Center for Consumer Freedom, a non-profit lobby group) serves as a front for the food industry. Its purpose is to "defend the right of adults and parents to choose how they live their lives, what they eat and drink, how they manage their finances and how they enjoy themselves."[11]

Coca Cola has been exposed in paying off three scientists to form the Global Energy Balance Network to pin the blame for obesity on lack of exercise. The soda industry has given more than $120 million USD to 96 health care organizations to promote their agendas but not a word about food industry regulation.[12]

The Sugar Research Foundation paid scientists to publish papers exonerating sugar and blaming fat for heart disease. Funded studies showing sugared beverages have no effect on weight gain, whereas independent studies showed just the opposite.[13]

The Academy of Nutrition and Dietetics accepted millions of dollars from food, pharmaceutical and agribusiness companies, had policies to provide favors in return, and invested in ultra-processed food company stocks, according to a study published in Public Health Nutrition.

The Academy of Nutrition and Dietetics says it is "the world's largest organization of nutrition and dietetics practitioners," representing "more than 112,000 credentialed practitioners" including registered dietitian nutritionists and other food and nutrition professionals. A study describes the "symbiotic relationship" between the Academy and corporations, and found the Academy acts as a "pro-industry voice" with policy positions that sometimes clash with its mission to improve health globally. The documents reveal a depressing chapter of corruption at this influential nutrition group. The study reveals that the Academy accepted more than $15 million from corporate and organizational contributors in the years 2011 and 2013-2017, according to its IRS forms 990.[14]

The International Food Information Council (IFIC) "promotes food and beverage company interests and undermines the accurate dissemination of scientific evidence related to diet and health," according to a study published in the *Journal Globalization and Health*. The IFIC is widely cited in the media as a source on consumer sentiment and matters related to food and health.

The study found that the IFIC often engages in consumer "preference shaping," which "includes the use of key opinion leaders and multimedia communications to promote narratives sympathetic to business interests." The group also is involved in "manufacturing doubt," which is using "specific evidence and rhetoric to create doubt about negative health impacts of specific foods or food groups. It works to protect food industry profits, not your health. The IFIC uses media outlets to preemptively counter information about the negative health impacts of added sugars and ultra-processed foods."

The IFIC was established to work closely with the food industry front group International Life Sciences Institute (ILSI), a group founded by former Coca-Cola senior vice president Alex Malaspina. Malaspina has described how the groups work together: "IFIC is kind of a sister entity to ILSI. ILSI generates the scientific facts and IFIC communicates them to the media and public."[15]

Medical practitioners and providers paid $26.8 billion over the past decade to settle federal allegations including fraud, bribery, and patient harm, a Reuters investigation found. Paying up means staying in business and, for some, avoiding prison. US prosecutors helped them do it.[16]

The Sugar Industry blocked research linking sucrose to heart disease and cancer from publication 50 *years* ago. The researchers at the University of California at San Francisco have uncovered data showing the Sugar Industry hid research linking sugar to cancer in 1968. New documents show the Sugar Association funded an animal experiment called Project 259 to evaluate sucrose's effects on cardiovascular health. But when the data showed a clear link between sucrose and poor heart health, they pulled the plug. The researchers say that, had this paper been published in 1968, it would have led to scrutiny and even regulation of sugar by the FDA.[17]

The Sugar Industry funded animal research in the 1960s that looked into the effects of sugar consumption on cardiovascular health—and then buried the data when it suggested that sugar could be harmful, according to newly released historical documents.[18]

50 YEARS AGO, SUGAR INDUSTRY QUIETLY PAID SCIENTISTS TO POINT BLAME AT FAT

In the 1960s, the Sugar Industry funded research that downplayed the risks of sugar and highlighted the hazards of fat, according to a newly published article in *JAMA Internal Medicine*. The article draws on internal documents to show that an industry group called the Sugar Research Foundation wanted to "refute" concerns about sugar's possible role in heart disease. The SRF then sponsored research by Harvard scientists that did just that. The result was published in the *New England Journal of Medicine* in 1967, with no disclosure of the Sugar Industry funding.

IT'S YOUR FAULT FOR NOT HAVING DISCIPLINE AND NOT EXERCISING

Blaming people for lack of exercise and discipline, not sugar, is what the Sugar Industry wants you to believe. Obesity is a behavior, a flaw in your character, a psychological aberration. And we don't pay for behavior. It's a lifestyle choice. Of course, there is no mention of how fructose actually lowers your energy and adds weight, which impedes exercise.

OBESITY IS WHAT IS KILLING YOU

You do not die from obesity, you die from the diseases that "travel" with obesity. Diabetes, hypertension, heart disease, cancer, dementia, and chronic kidney disease are what kills you, and sugar consumption is the primary link to these diseases.[19]

THE DIET WARS

Diets are promoted to be the solution, but if they worked there would not be a diet industry.

Can you see how average people in the US and this world today, who often struggle to find truthful news, are having a hard time knowing the truth about sugar? With this much money, power and influence lined up against us, it makes a mockery of the term "informed consent." At least today, tobacco smokers, drug users (other than sugar addicts) and alcoholics all have informed consent. They have an informed choice to make. But we cannot say the same for sugar addicts.

CHAPTER 8
FOLLOW THE MONEY AND YE SHALL KNOW THE TRUTH

I realize some readers may not be religious, may have a different faith, or no faith at all, but I do want to make some points about money from a human and spiritual perspective.

Just over 2200 years ago there was a very famous person who preached to large audiences and performed a number of miracles (or some would believe, great magic tricks). People have varying opinions whether he was the son of God, a prophet, a magician, or simply a great public speaker. Most people think he mainly preached about love, but upon closer examination, he spoke more about avarice, greed and the dangers of loving money. I personally think he was correct in his message and that following the money, today, is always a sound idea in order to know the truth.

Sure enough, after doing a bit of research on this subject it's almost alarming how much Jesus talked about money. He discussed the topic of money more often than he spoke of faith and prayer. Eleven of his 40 parables were about money or used money as a way to teach spiritual truths. As far as the New Testament is concerned, greed is considered to be more of a threat for the ability to follow Christ than lust.

Avarice, money, and greed are timely topics. It is increasingly common today to hear people talking about greed growing out of control as a fundamental cause of our world's woes—economic or otherwise. We continue to be troubled that some make millions in bonuses and salaries while lower-level employees and workers are living paycheck to paycheck. Garish profits are being made without concern for negative downstream effects. Greed seems to have no limits or shame.

Examples of major industries driven by greed that may cause more harm than good:

- Sugar Industry
- Military-industrial complex
- Tobacco
- Alcohol and drugs
- Gambling
- One could argue credit card companies, Wall Street bankers, social media, etc.

By following the money, I mean who is making the money, how are they doing it, are they doing it legally and transparently and is that money helping or hurting society? This is very important to understand in order for each of us to have a healthy skepticism about the information and news that we receive, which may have ulterior financial incentives and influences that result in us being misinformed or lied to.

CAN OUR TRUSTED SOURCES OF INFORMATION BE TRUSTED?

Should we blindly trust all of our major governmental and corporate institutions?

Military-Industrial Complex

During his farewell address in January 1961, President Eisenhower warned Americans and the Congress about the dangers of the military-industrial complex. The military-industrial complex is the close relationship between the US military and the giant corporations that built its weapons. America was expecting Eisenhower to rail about the perils of the cold war, nuclear arms, Communism and the threat of Russian expansion and domination. But no, he was warning us about the military-industrial complex. He saw the tremendous buildup and influence of the lobbyists and money interests, and their effect upon the Congress and news media. Flash forward to today and the Center for Responsive Politics noted the defense sector spent more than $120,000,000 dollars on lobbying efforts in 2021 alone.

Let's move back to Oct 1967. I was in San Antonio Texas sitting in a training class during my Air Force Officer's Training School (OTS) boot camp learning about the justification for the Vietnam war. It had to do with Nixon's domino theory and stopping Communism. The logical explanation was that if Vietnam falls, then Cambodia and Laos would be next, then Thailand, Singapore, and Indonesia. Then New Zealand and Australia, etc. Sort of like a bunch of lined-up dominos collapsing. What was not mentioned was that Vietnam's biggest threat and enemy over many centuries was Red China, not the West. Vietnam just wanted their country back with some type of initial socialist government, which in time, as we have discovered, became a very strong capitalist competitor. But basically, the US government was delivering an important message that, by intent or ignorance, was omitting a very important point: the domino theory was BS and Vietnam was not going to be a threat to anyone. Nor did Vietnam wish to be a part of China.

The US military-industrial complex, which consisted of defense contractors and whose political supporters are now referred to as Neocons, lobbied the government to increase military spending and to continue providing military aid to Vietnam. The war in Vietnam was a very profitable business for the military-industrial complex. Defense contractors such as Boeing, General Electric, Northrop, Lockheed Martin, Raytheon, etc., earned billions of dollars from supplying the military with weapons, aircraft, and other equipment. They lobbied the government to continue the war to maintain their profits, even as public opinion turned against the war and the cost in lives and expenditures increased.

In Stephen Kinzer's book *Overthrow*, he basically covers the 28 wars and military operations and excursions conducted by the United States since 1898. In hindsight, one could argue that the US should not have been engaged in 24 of those wars and operations, including Vietnam, Iraq, Afghanistan, and now Ukraine. Some of those excursions were more about protecting business interests who wanted to get control of their banana plantations in some small Central American country. But most of these wars and operations were all about money, whether it be protecting business interests or simply developing and supplying new weapon systems and buying armaments to fight such wars. You can rest assured that the military-industrial complex had its fingerprints on many of these wars and operations while being protected and promoted by the Congress, lobbyists, and advertising influence in the news media. You can also be assured that the military industry needs wars to make big profits.

So, what does this have to do with sugar? Please allow me some grace and read on as it is very important that you start the process of following the money and how it is very possible that you are being misled, or even lied to, even today, about sugar and processed foods.

Big Tobacco

This is another example of needing to follow the money and is covered in more detail in Chapter 16. Tobacco companies had free reign for more than half a century in the US, where they and their lobbyists splashed money across the Congress, news media, and even the medical community. Once informed consent began in the 1960s and 70s, and Big Tobacco lawsuits took place in the 80s, it still took 30 years to reduce tobacco smoking in the US from 42% to 12%. If you follow the money, you will see how Big Tobacco misled and lied to the American public while keeping Congress and the news media under its heel. Follow the money some more and you see that Big Tobacco, once they saw pending negative tobacco legislation, were on the losing end of multi-billion-dollar lawsuits and public awareness turning more and more negative, Big Tobacco decided to take a protective step, by making huge investments in processed food companies. In this way they could move their wares and profits from nicotine addiction to sugar addiction.

MAJOR CORPORATE FRAUDS

Since the year 2000 there have been ten major corporations that were fraudulent in pulling the wool over our eyes to the tune of more than $1 trillion in losses to the public, which never saw it coming, because of lobbying and influence in the news media and Congress. The general public was being lied to or misinformed.

Wall Street and Subprime Mortgages

All of us can remember the biggest crash since the Great Depression: the subprime mortgage crisis of 2007-2008. Many books such as *The Big Short: Inside the Doomsday Machine*, by Michael Lewis; *Too Big to Fail: The Inside Story of How Wall Street and Washington Fought to Save the Financial System—and Themselves*, by Andrew Ross Sorkin; and *All the Devils Are Here: The Hidden History of the Financial Crisis*, by Bethany McLean and Joe Nocera, all chronicle the lies, corruption, and cozy regulatory relationships of Wall Street and the US government.

The US Sick Care System

Also called healthcare, this system makes money by treating patients, not through preventative medicine. If all patients suddenly got more healthy all the hospitals, health insurance companies, PBMs and Big Pharma would see profits reduced greatly. But when you look under the lid of the US healthcare system, you will find that less than 2% of expenditures are for preventative medicine and fewer than 1% of doctors are trained in nutrition. Doctors are trained to treat sick people by design. They are purposely not trained in preventative medicine and nutrition. Thus they are treating the symptoms of sugar addiction, not the cause.

Currently, the United States spends approximately $4.3 trillion on healthcare, which accounts for around 18.3% of the country's gross domestic product (GDP). This figure includes spending on healthcare services, medical equipment, and pharmaceuticals, as well as public health activities and research.

Despite the high level of spending, the US does not have the best health outcomes compared to other developed countries. Life expectancy in the US is lower than in many other high-income countries, and the US has higher rates of chronic diseases such as diabetes and obesity.

Remember, Big Pharma employs 1,834 lobbyists to run through the halls of Congress with handouts, trips, and money for re-election campaigns. Big Pharma representatives visit thousands of doctors' offices daily in the US handing out their free samples, weekend golfing trips, and Caribbean vacations for doctors achieving their prescription quotas. The next major influence on the American public is the news media, TV, cable, and newspapers. Can you guess who is the biggest advertiser today in those media? Yes, you guessed it: it is Big Pharma.

For those living in the United States this has come to be accepted as normal, but only in the United States and New Zealand is Big Pharma allowed to advertise pharmaceutical products directly to the consumer. Perhaps one should wonder why 181 countries do not allow this?

Let me make one final point, which is what came from the NIH during the pandemic. We know that Big Pharma has a lot of clout with the NIH, the CDC and the FDA. Therefore, I was not surprised by the questionable information stream that came out of Washington DC as Covid emerged and the pandemic went into full swing. No more gyms, no more exercise, no more sunshine, staying at home eating more convenience foods was the advice of the NIH, all of it wrong as will be seen later in Chapter 15, "Covid: The Lost Opportunity." This edict was followed by an almost mandatory requirement to be vaccinated with basically untested Covid vaccines that would prevent one from getting Covid. Later this was amended to say the vaccine would stop the prevention of Covid. This was followed by the message that if you get vaccinated, you won't get Covid again. Finally, that Covid immunity is better than natural immunity. All of this in hindsight ended up being false, and we do not know how much of this was due to ignorance, misinformation or lies. But we do know there was big money behind it as seen in the profits by Pfizer, J&J, Moderna and other vaccine makers. It was almost mind boggling to look at Moderna's stock price chart moving from $14 to $440 during the pandemic.

On January 10, *Time* and *CNN* reported that President Trump was appointing RFK Jr. to be the vaccine czar. His new responsibilities, Kennedy said, included making sure "we have scientific integrity in the vaccine process for efficacy and safety effects." He also stressed that "everybody ought to be able to be assured that the vaccines we have [are] as safe as they can possibly be." Finally, he added that Trump "is very pro-vaccine, as am I."

Within 48 hours, the appointment was rescinded and perhaps coincidentally, Pfizer donated $1 million USD to the Trump campaign and had two of its executives appointed to key positions in the NIH and FDA. A coincidence? You decide.

Now let's turn to the real reason for writing this chapter, which is this: maybe we are not getting the straight skinny from our government, the news media, our doctors, and other key trusted information sources for maintaining our good health. The healthcare business in the US alone is a $4.3 trillion annual business, which is a lot of money by anybody's standards. In fact, the expenditures for US healthcare exceed the GDPs of 181 countries and is only exceeded by the GDPs of China and Japan.

Dr. Robert Lustig, an accredited MD, endocrinologist, and now attorney, has written several illuminating books (*Fat Chance*, *Metabolical* and *The Hacking of the American Mind*), which tell the real story as well as anybody. Dr. Lustig, who is discussed in more detail in Chapter 11, covers in detail that approximately 75% of our healthcare problems are due to our consumption of sugar, sugar-added products, and processed foods. He mentions specifically the links to heart disease, cancer, diabetes, chronic kidney disease, fatty liver, and Alzheimer's. If you take 75% of $4.3 trillion USD, that is a big number. For those of you who are mathematically impaired, that is $3.2 trillion USD. That expenditure ties it with India for the world's fifth largest GDP.

On top of this, the US government does not subsidize alcohol, tobacco or drugs—just sugar. You would think somebody at one of our so-called health agencies would object to creating incentives to grow sugar?

A CURRENT EXAMPLE OF US GOVERNMENT CENSORSHIP

On May 5, 2022, the attorneys general of Louisiana and Missouri filed suit in the US District Court for the Western District of Louisiana, alleging the federal government coerced, coordinated, and colluded with social media platforms to censor First Amendment protected speech online. Defendants included the Biden White House and nine other agencies, including the FBI and parts of DHS.

On July 4, 2023, the district court granted most of the plaintiffs' request for a preliminary injunction, which enjoined the government and specifically named federal officials, including White House officials, from (1) communicating in any way with social media companies to censor or suppress protected speech on their platforms, or (2) using third-party organizations to accomplish the same. The court's decision exempted security threats and other illegal activity in its 155-page ruling.

COULD OUR GOVERNMENT BE CENSORING INFORMATION ABOUT WHAT WE EAT?

By now you should be keenly aware, when you follow the Big Money, that it should make you suspicious and that you may not find the truth. Follow the money and ask yourself, "Am I 100% confident that I have been given all the facts and that I am being told the truth about what I am eating and drinking?"

CHAPTER 9
SUGAR SCIENCE FOR DUMMIES
HOW SUGAR KILLS US SOFTLY

L et's get one simple fact understood: *there is no human requirement for sugar.* You could almost say it is a recreational drug with devastating long-term consequences, hence the title, *Killing You Softly*, could have also been *Killing You Slowly* or *Killing You Sweetly*.

In previous chapters we saw the origins and history of sugar, as well as who makes up the Sugar Industry. I gave my definition of the Sugar Industry as anybody who profits from sugar in any way. Now I want to inform you of what happens when you put sugar into your mouth, as well as high-fructose corn syrup and processed foods, sugar's unhealthy cousins. They basically all do the same thing— destroy your good health.

You know my story of how my life got saved by a miracle and how I discovered that the cause of my metabolic syndrome was sugar. What you do not know is the origins of my research that led to my conclusion that sugar was not only killing me softly, but was killing the entire world.

As you know, my discovery process started after I had read my first anti-sugar book, *Sugar Crush* and experienced my amazing transformation after my 21-day detox. Shortly thereafter, I viewed a Dr. Robert Lustig YouTube video of a sugar lecture he gave to a graduate school class at the University of California that has now gone viral with more than 25 million viewings. When you think about this, it is astounding that a long, technical, complex student lecture could garner this many views. In case you wish to know the biochemistry of what happens when sugar enters your body you can see it at this link:

https://www.youtube.com/watch?v=dBnniua6-oM or just Google, "Sugar, the Bitter Truth."

This video motivated me to further investigate, which led me to read the following books:

1. *Sugar Crush*, by Richard Jacoby MD – the original book that was the catalyst that saved my life.
2. *Fat Chance*, by Robert H. Lustig MD, MSL – one of the most complete anti-sugar books ever written.
3. *The Case Against Sugar*, by Gary Taubes – a layperson's research guide to the truth about sugar.
4. *The Sugar Fix*, by Richard J. Johnson MD – a well-written treatise about how sugar makes it impossible to lose weight, amongst other things.
5. *The Salt Fix*, by James DiNicolantonio MD – clears up misperception about salt and high blood pressure when it is sugar that is the leading problem.
6. *Pure, White and Deadly*, by John Yudkin – the first major book to expose the perils of consuming sugar.
7. *Sugar Blues*, by William Dufty – shows how a revitalizing, sugar-free diet can not only change lives, but quite possibly save them.
8. *The Hacking of the American Mind*, by Robert H. Lustig, MD, MSL - ties sugar to the corrupting of American society and links to depression and suicide.
9. *Fat and Cholesterol Don't Cause Heart Attacks and Statins Are Not the Solution*, by Dr. Paul J. Rosch. Maybe it's the sugar that is the problem?
10. *Fast Food Genocide*, by Joel Fuhrman MD - how fast food is wreaking havoc on our health.
11. *Sweet Poison – Why Sugar Makes Us Fat*, by David Gillespie - just like the title says.

12. *Drop Acid*, by David Perlmutter, MD - elevated uric acid levels lie at the root of many pervasive health conditions, but doctors often remain unaware of this connection.

13. *Spring Chicken*, by Bill Gifford - a humorous but insightful synopsis of current ways to stay younger and healthier.

14. *The Fat Switch*, by Richard J. Johnson MD - how mankind's survival switch of 10 million years ago has now turned into a fat switch due to sugar consumption.

15. *Death by Food Pyramid*, by Denise Minger - nicely done and shows how the US government stacked the unhealthy diet cards against us.

16. *The Plant Paradox*, by Steven R. Gundry, MD - a thought-provoking book with some different slants on eating real food.

17. *The pH Miracle*, by Robert O. Young, PhD and Shelley Redford Young - how acidic or alkaline your blood is (pH levels) affects your health and is controlled by diet.

18. *How Not to Die*, by Michael Greger, MD, FACLM - dives into nutrition science, providing overwhelming compelling evidence for food as medicine.

19. *Keto Diet*, by Josh Axe MD - an informative look at the keto diet and ketosis.

20. *Eat Rich, Live Long*, by Jeffry Gerber MD and Ivor Cummins - take control of your health, lose weight, prevent disease, and enjoy a long and healthy life.

21. *Metabolical*, by Robert H. Lustig MD, MSL - how processed food has impacted and ruined our health, economy, and environment over the past 50 years.

22. *Life Force*, by Tony Robbins, Peter Diamandis MD, and Robert Hariri MD, PhD - an up-to-date summary of the latest advances in anti-aging and preventive medicine.

23. *Lifespan, Why We Age and Why We Don't Have To*, by David A. Sinclair, PhD – if you wish to live longer then this anti-aging book is a must-read .

Besides these books I have watched hundreds of hours of videos and podcasts from such informed luminaries as:

- Peter Attia, MD
- Andrew Huberman, MD
- Peter Diamandis, MD
- Robert H. Lustig, MD
- Robert J. Johnson, MD
- Aseem Malhorta, MD
- David Perlmutter, MD
- Joel Fuhrman, MD
- Florence Christophers - Kick Sugar Summit series
- Mike Collins - Quit Sugar Summit series

In addition to all the books, podcasts and hundreds of articles and research reports, interestingly they all said the same thing: sugar is destroying your health and needs to be reduced and/or eliminated from your diet.

WHAT IS FOOD?

There are two important definitions to discuss. A food is defined as a substance that provides nutrition and promotes growth, while a poison is a substance that promotes illness or even death. Which of these definitions do sugar and processed foods fit? If you think sugar and processed foods are actually food, then the last 10-20 years of your life are not going to be much fun.

A simple way to look at anything that you put into your mouth is this: does this substance protect my liver and feed my gut? Those foods that satisfy both precepts are healthy, those that do neither are poison, and those that do only one are bad for your health.[1]

SUGAR BASICS

With all of this in mind, please be assured that I am in a position to teach sugar science to the reader. We thus will start with the basics.

Sugar is composed of glucose and fructose. The Sugar Industry will have you believe that sugar is necessary for life and that you cannot live without glucose. Well, they got half of that right. You cannot live without glucose as our cells need glucose to live. The Sugar Industry likes to keep you confused by blurring the distinction of glucose (blood sugar) with sucrose (sugar which is composed of glucose and fructose). In summary, glucose is body fuel, while sucrose is body poison.

There are two things that our friends in the Sugar Industry do not really tell us or emphasize. The first is that there are other healthy sources of glucose (other than sugar and processed foods) such as the following:

- **Many fruits** contain natural sugars, including glucose. Examples include blueberries, melons, mangos, bananas, apples, grapes, and oranges. Basically, all fruit contains essential vitamins, minerals, and fiber, making them a healthy choice.
- **Certain vegetables** like sweet potatoes, carrots, and beets contain natural sugars, including glucose. They are also rich in fiber, antioxidants, and other beneficial nutrients.
- **Whole grains** like oats, brown rice, quinoa, and whole wheat are excellent sources of complex carbohydrates, which are broken down into glucose in the body. These grains provide a steady release of energy and are more nutritious than refined grains.
- **Legumes:** Lentils, chickpeas, black beans, and other legumes are not only rich in protein and fiber, but also provide a good amount of glucose. They offer a slow and sustained release of energy due to their complex carbohydrate content.
- **Honey:** Honey is a natural sweetener that contains glucose along with fructose and other sugars. It also contains antioxidants and antibacterial properties. However, it should be consumed in moderation due to its sugar content.
- **Dairy products:** Milk and yogurt contain lactose, a sugar that is broken down into glucose and galactose in the body.

Dairy products also provide calcium, protein, and other essential nutrients.

- Some types of **dietary fiber** can be fermented by gut bacteria to produce short-chain fatty acids, including small amounts of glucose.
- Our bodies can also convert other nutrients like **proteins and fats** into glucose through various metabolic processes.
- The liver can make glucose from triglycerides in dietary or body fat or from amino acids; in other words, it converts your fat cells into glucose, a great natural way to shed those excess pounds.

Let's discuss what happens with sugar's two components: glucose and fructose.

Fructose, the worst of the two, is a type of sugar commonly found in fruits, honey, and some processed foods and soft drinks. It is metabolized differently than glucose in the body.

Fructose is absorbed into the bloodstream through the walls of the small intestine with the help of specific transport proteins. Once absorbed, fructose is primarily metabolized in the liver. Unlike glucose, which is metabolized in various tissues, fructose metabolism is largely confined to the liver. By the way, the liver is the only organ that metabolizes poisons.

The next six paragraphs are for those readers who passed their organic chemistry and biochemistry classes in college. Feel free to skip these paragraphs or perhaps plow on so you can try to explain this to your possibly overweight nextdoor neighbor couch potato.

Fructose is converted into fructose-1-phosphate by an enzyme called fructokinase. This step requires the consumption of ATP (adenosine triphosphate), which is an energy-rich molecule, fructose-1-phosphate. This is a very important point to note because by consuming ATP to metabolize any poison (sugar, in this case) you are actually using/lowering your energy. This affects your entire body including your brain.

Fructose-1-phosphate is then further broken down into glyceraldehyde and dihydroxyacetone phosphate by an enzyme called aldolase

B. Glyceraldehyde and dihydroxyacetone phosphate can enter the glycolytic pathway, a metabolic process that converts glucose or its metabolites into pyruvate.

One unique aspect of fructose metabolism is its tendency to be readily converted into fatty acids. Fructose can be used as a precursor for de novo lipogenesis, which is the synthesis of new fatty acids. Excess fructose consumption, especially in the form of added sugars, will contribute to increased fat storage and to the development of fatty liver.

Fructose metabolism also leads to the production of uric acid. Fructose metabolism increases the production of purine nucleotides, which are broken down into uric acid. Elevated uric acid levels are associated with conditions such as gout and metabolic syndrome.

It's important to note that excessive consumption of fructose, particularly in the form of added sugars like high-fructose corn syrup, has been linked to negative health effects such as weight gain, insulin resistance, metabolic syndrome, increased risk of fatty liver disease, and a myriad of other diseases.

CLEARING UP THE FRUIT MYSTERY

Fruits, which contain fructose along with essential vitamins, minerals, antioxidants, and fiber, are an important component of a healthy diet and provide numerous health benefits. So how can this be if fruit is a source of fructose?

Please note: It's the Fiber

I want to clear this up as I know it is in the back of your mind and I do not want you to be alarmed as you read about all the bad things that fructose does to us. The key is the fiber.

When you eat fruit (not fruit juice or smoothies), you are consuming fiber. Fiber is composed of both soluble and insoluble fiber. Fiber is our friend as it performs two incredibly valuable functions.

First, it creates a lattice network in our stomach and esophageal linings that protect us from absorbing the fructose into our bloodstream and attacking our livers. It basically slows or prevents the absorption, thus pushing it down to our gut biomes.

Secondly, it performs that very valuable function of feeding our gut biomes, the home of a trillion bacteria that need to eat or they do bad things like not producing serotonin, our happiness hormone, or munching down on our intestinal linings (leaky gut), causing IBD (irritable bowel syndrome), Crohn's disease, diarrhea, and a myriad of other damaging things.

You have heard the expression "happy wife, happy life." Well, even more important, a healthy gut means a happy healthy life.

ALCOHOL: SUGAR'S OTHER INSIDIOUS FRIEND

I grew up in a military family and I can tell you that our military likes to party. Drinking is the norm, so it did not take me long to get into that rat race and I wish I could take back the majority of the drinking that I did in my younger years as I know that it has limited my life span, health, and pocketbook.

The problem is alcohol has ethanol as its featured ingredient and although it does not convert into sugar, it is processed in a similar manner. About 10% of ethanol is metabolized in the stomach and intestines (called the first-pass effect) while another 10% is metabolized in the brain (where we get our buzz). However, the majority of alcohol metabolism occurs in the liver where enzymes work to convert ethanol into acetaldehyde, which is a toxic and potentially harmful substance. Acetaldehyde is further metabolized by ALDH into acetate, a less toxic substance. Finally, acetate is broken down into carbon dioxide and water, which are harmless byproducts that can be easily eliminated from the body.

Alcohol metabolism occurs at a relatively constant rate, typically around one standard drink per hour. Consuming alcohol faster than the liver can metabolize it can lead to an accumulation of acetaldehyde, causing the symptoms of intoxication.

Various factors can influence alcohol metabolism, such as age, sex, body weight, liver health, and the presence of other drugs or medications. Additionally, different individuals may have variations in the activity of alcohol-metabolizing enzymes, which can impact how they respond to alcohol consumption.

Excessive alcohol consumption over time can lead to liver damage and other health issues, as the liver has a limited capacity to metabolize alcohol. Therefore, it's essential to consume alcohol in moderation and be aware of its potential effects on the body.

Some studies have shown that a little bit of alcohol can be good for you as it can raise your good cholesterol, HDL, and promote better endothelial function, which is essential for healthy blood vessels. Moderate alcohol intake has been associated with reduced blood clot formation, which can help prevent certain types of cardiovascular events.

My weakness is red wine, especially Malbecs. Red wine contains antioxidants like resveratrol and flavonoids, which can help neutralize harmful free radicals in the body, potentially reducing oxidative stress and inflammation that contribute to heart disease. Moderate red wine consumption is the key here, as excessive alcohol consumption can have serious negative effects on health.

My love for red wine comes more from how it complements food and how much I enjoy it with a meal. My research shows that a glass of red wine with a meal 2-4 times a week should not impair my health and may actually be a plus, as noted above.

Each person needs to do his or her own research on this subject, but be advised that booze is no friend of your liver, and just like sugar and processed foods, can lead to chronic disease.

NOW BACK TO THE BAD FRUCTOSE NEWS

High fructose intake contributes to weight gain and obesity. Fructose is metabolized differently than glucose and has been shown to be more readily converted into fatty acids, which contribute to increased fat storage. Consuming large amounts of fructose, especially in the form of sugary beverages and processed foods, will contribute to excess calorie intake and weight gain.

High fructose consumption is associated with insulin resistance, a condition in which cells become less responsive to the effects of insulin. Insulin resistance is a precursor to type 2 diabetes. Excessive fructose intake will lead to impaired glucose metabolism and dysregu-lation of insulin levels.

Consuming excessive amounts of fructose, particularly in the form of added sugars, will contribute to the development of non-alcoholic fatty liver disease (NAFLD). The metabolism of fructose in the liver will result in increased fat accumulation and inflammation in the liver, potentially leading to liver damage.

High fructose intake will elevate blood triglyceride levels, which are a type of fat in the bloodstream. Elevated triglyceride levels are associated with an increased risk of cardiovascular disease.

"Fructose is not bad because of its calories, but because it has effects on liver metabolism to make it worse at burning fat. As a result, adding fructose to the diet makes the liver store more fat, and this is bad for the liver and bad for whole body metabolism."[2]

Dr. Richard Johnson has noted that fructose is the only nutrient that actually reduces the ATP in our body, so it actually reduces the energy we use, which, in turn, drives our fat switch as we become lethargic when ATP levels fall inside the cell. It is like an alarm signal. It stimu-lates hunger and thirst, like it did 20 million years ago, creating a foraging response. This is where we get our food cravings.

Fructose metabolism leads to increased production of uric acid, which can contribute to the development of gout, a form of arthritis. Elevated uric acid levels are also associated with an increased risk of kidney stones and metabolic syndrome. Personally, my uric acid levels were always above the upper suggested range, yet my doctors never said a word about this and seemed to be more worried about other things like my high blood pressure and my cholesterol. Since quitting sugar and processed foods, my uric acid levels are, for the first time, in range. Also, during my sugar-eating days I had two kidney stone attacks and also had Bell's Palsy (an inflammation of the F 7 cranial nerve, which makes your face go numb). Since quitting sugar there have been no recurrences.

Hopefully, by now you know that fructose found in sugar, processed foods, high-fructose corn syrup (HFCS) and soft drinks is a definite *no-no*. Many popular soft drinks will have HFCS added along with sugar. Also, catsups, sauces, candy bars, and some processed foods will have HFCS as an ingredient. When a label says high-fructose corn syrup, HFCS, corn syrup, then do this: *run!*

EXCESS GLUCOSE CAN ALSO BE BAD NEWS

As noted previously there are plenty of ways for humans to consume vital glucose, and all of them are healthy and found in real food. But sugar and processed foods also provide glucose along with its dastardly cousin, fructose. Because sugar is so habit-forming and we end up overeating it in our processed foods, fast foods, sweets and snacks, excess amounts of glucose are received that the body does not need and which insulin will remove and store as fat. We will discuss insulin a little later.

Glucose metabolism is a complex process that occurs in our bodies to obtain energy from glucose, a simple sugar. Glucose metabolism begins with glycolysis, which takes place in the cytoplasm of cells. In this process, one molecule of glucose is broken down into two molecules of pyruvate. This step does not require oxygen and results in a small amount of ATP (adenosine triphosphate) production. If oxygen is present, the pyruvate molecules produced in glycolysis enter the mitochondria of cells. There, each pyruvate is converted into acetyl-CoA, generating a molecule of carbon dioxide and one molecule of NADH (nicotinamide adenine dinucleotide).

Acetyl-CoA enters the citric acid cycle, also known as the Krebs cycle, which takes place in the mitochondria. In this cycle, acetyl-CoA is further broken down, releasing more carbon dioxide and generating additional molecules of NADH and FADH2 (flavin adenine dinucleotide).

NADH and FADH2 produced in previous steps enter the electron transport chain, located in the inner mitochondrial membrane. Through a series of redox reactions, these molecules donate electrons, generating a flow of protons (H+) across the membrane. This flow of protons drives ATP synthesis, producing a large amount of ATP, which is used as the primary energy source for various cellular processes. This is all good and critical for sustaining life.

If there is an excess of glucose in the bloodstream, the body employs mechanisms to regulate blood glucose levels and prevent them from becoming too high. The main hormone involved in this process is insulin, which is released by the pancreas. When blood glucose levels rise, the pancreas secretes insulin into the bloodstream. Insulin acts as a signal to various cells, particularly in the liver, muscle, and adipose tissue (fat cells).

Insulin facilitates the uptake of glucose by cells, particularly in muscle and adipose tissue. The cells have insulin receptors on their surface that bind to insulin, triggering the translocation of glucose transporters (GLUT4) to the cell membrane. This allows glucose to enter the cells from the bloodstream, reducing blood glucose levels.

In the liver and muscles, excess glucose is converted into glycogen through a process called glycogenesis. Insulin promotes glycogen synthesis and storage, allowing excess glucose to be stored for later use. When there is excess glucose beyond the storage capacity of glycogen, insulin promotes the conversion of glucose into fatty acids through lipogenesis. These fatty acids are then stored as triglycerides in adipose tissue, leading to fat accumulation.

In summary, when there is excess glucose in the bloodstream, insulin is released to facilitate the uptake of glucose by cells, promote glycogen synthesis, suppress gluconeogenesis, and stimulate fat storage. These mechanisms work together to regulate blood glucose levels and maintain them within a normal range, but please notice the last item: stimulate fat storage.

INSULIN, FRIEND OR FOE?

Insulin is an essential hormone for regulating blood glucose levels and facilitating glucose uptake by cells. However, in certain situations, there can be potential harms associated with insulin. Here are a few examples.

One of the potential risks of using insulin or having excess insulin in the body is hypoglycemia, which is low blood sugar levels. If too much insulin is administered or released in response to high carbohydrate intake, it can cause blood sugar levels to drop below normal. Hypoglycemia can lead to symptoms such as dizziness, confusion, weakness, and, in severe cases, even loss of consciousness or seizures. It is important to carefully manage insulin dosages and monitor blood sugar levels to avoid hypoglycemia.

Insulin promotes the storage of excess glucose as fat in adipose tissue through lipogenesis. This means that individuals who require insulin injections or have conditions that result in insulin resistance (e.g., type 2 diabetes) will experience weight gain or find it more challenging to lose weight.

Prolonged exposure to high levels of insulin, as seen in conditions like obesity or type 2 diabetes, can lead to insulin resistance. Insulin resistance occurs when cells become less responsive to the effects of insulin, resulting in higher insulin levels required to achieve the desired glucose uptake. This can contribute to further metabolic dysregulation, impaired glucose control, and increased risk of developing type 2 diabetes and other associated health complications related to chronic disease.

Insulin's role in promoting lipogenesis and inhibiting lipolysis (the breakdown of stored fats) can lead to elevated levels of triglycerides in the blood. High levels of triglycerides are associated with an increased risk of cardiovascular disease.

It's important to note that insulin is a vital hormone for maintaining glucose homeostasis, and the potential harms mentioned above are associated with excessive or imbalanced insulin levels.

Insulin release is primarily triggered by elevated blood glucose levels. When you consume food, especially carbohydrates, the carbohydrates are broken down into glucose during digestion. As a result, the concentration of glucose in the bloodstream increases, thus prompting the release of insulin into the bloodstream. Insulin acts as a hormone that helps regulate glucose metabolism throughout the body.

When you consume sugar, especially refined sugars or high-glycemic carbohydrates, it causes a rapid increase in blood glucose levels. This is known as a blood sugar spike or blood sugar surge. In response to the increased blood glucose levels, the pancreas releases more insulin. Now you may be on your way to diabetes and chronic disease.

The bottom line is that sugar turns our insulin friend into a foe.

INTRODUCING LEPTIN: OUR HUNGER-CONTROL COP

Insulin and leptin are two separate hormones with distinct roles in the body, and they can interact with each other in complex ways. While insulin does not directly inhibit leptin, there is overwhelming evidence to suggest that insulin levels can influence leptin signaling and sensitivity.

Leptin is a hormone primarily produced by adipose tissue (fat cells) and plays a role in regulating energy balance and appetite. Leptin levels generally correlate with body fat stores, and higher levels of leptin are associated with decreased appetite and increased energy expenditure.

Insulin modulates the production and signaling of leptin in several ways. Firstly, insulin can directly stimulate the production and release of leptin from adipose tissue. Higher insulin levels, such as in conditions of insulin resistance or obesity, can lead to elevated leptin levels.

Insulin resistance, a condition where cells become less responsive to the effects of insulin, can also affect leptin signaling. In cases of insulin resistance, it is common to observe a phenomenon called "leptin resistance," where the body becomes less sensitive to the appetite-suppressing effects of leptin. This can lead to disrupted appetite regulation and contribute to weight gain. In obesity, despite high levels of leptin being present in circulation, individuals may still experience diminished sensitivity to its effects, leading to a condition known as "leptin resistance." Leptin resistance thus contributes to increased appetite, overeating, and difficulty in losing weight. One might also call this sugar cravings.

In summary, leptin which acts like your satiety police officer, who, instead of telling you that you are full, is now sleeping at the post, thanks to insulin, so you do not even know that you are full. Thus, you are still hungry and overeat unhealthy food that is making you sicker. This never-ending addictive unhealthy eating cycle of sugar-laced processed foods leads to more chronic disease and, in the case of the United States, to being one of the most unhealthy countries in the world. The rest of the world should take notice, as you are next!

CHAPTER 10
THE DISTURBING TRENDS OF SUGAR CONSUMPTION

S ugar consumption of all types has gone from seven pounds per person per year in 1900 to more than 220 pounds per person per year on average today. This by itself is the foundation of sickness and disease that guarantees conventional medicine perpetual multi trillion-dollar annual sales and profits. Let's examine some of the negatives so you can appreciate the scope of the soft-killing, long-term effects caused by sugar and processed-food consumption (remember that processed foods have added sugar and/ or convert to sugar).

SUGAR REDUCES LIFE EXPECTANCY

The United States spends a whopping 18% of its GDP on healthcare. That's twice as much as most other industrialized countries. Yet we hardly receive a decent return on investment. America has the highest maternal mortality rates and the shortest life expectancy among all developed countries. Why is this?

Some recent studies and headlines on this topic include:

Much of the capital we invest in healthcare is going towards administrative costs involved with insurance; defensive care (when doctors order exams in fear of litigation); and towards the upkeep of a fragmented system, with an unparalleled number of different payers, billing staff, and specialized providers, resulting in significant inefficiencies and a lack of coordination.[1]

In a large review of 73 meta-analyses—which included 8,601 studies—high consumption of added sugar was associated with significantly higher risks of 45 negative health outcomes, including diabetes, gout, obesity, high blood pressure, heart attack, stroke, cancer, asthma, tooth decay, depression, and early death.[2]

Regular consumption of sugary drinks heightens the risk not only of tooth decay, obesity, fatty liver disease, and type 2 diabetes, but also of heart disease and premature death.[3]

Noncommunicable diseases (NCDs), including heart disease, stroke, cancer, diabetes, and chronic lung disease, are collectively responsible for 74% of all deaths worldwide.[4]

"Dr. Richard Johnson notes that fructose turns out to have been meant to be this wonderful system for survival, but in our culture with the amount of sugar in foods that we are eating (that either provide sugar or can be turned into fructose), this pathway has become hazardous."[5]

PROCESSED FOODS: SUGAR'S SECRET FRIEND AND SUBTLE KILLER

I really want you to consider quitting eating processed foods. I know, they are everywhere, convenient and so hard to resist. But let's see if we can motivate you, so read on.

Processed Foods Have Led to a Lack of Real Food in Our Supermarkets

At issue is the explosive growth in a broad class of food products that are not merely processed in the conventional sense to lengthen shelf life, but are also often modified to maximize flavor, visual appeal, texture, odor, and the speed with which they are digested. These foods are made by deconstructing natural food into its chemical constituents, modifying them and recombining them into new forms that bear little resemblance to anything found in nature. So radically are they altered that nutrition scientists have given them a new name: ultra-processed. The bottom line is ultra processed foods make us fat and unhealthy.

Being severely overweight has never been so dangerous. During the COVID-19 pandemic, Americans who are obese, without any other risk factors, were hospitalized at three times the rate of those who weren't, by some estimates. When combined with other diet-related health conditions, such as cardiovascular disease and diabetes, obesity raises the risk of hospitalization sixfold and the risk of death twelvefold.

The implications are worrisome. Half of American adults now have diabetes or pre-diabetes, three quarters of adults are overweight, and about 100 million, or 42%, are obese by the standards of the Centers for Disease Control and Prevention (CDC). Among children between two and five years old, one in ten are already obese. Among teens, that number is one in five.

Our food, in other words, is literally killing us. Food companies have tricked our brains into making us complicit, and our elected officials are complicit, too. What's needed is a better understanding of exactly how processed foods make us sick and a public reckoning with Big Food's role in the nation's health crisis. So far, policymakers have shown little appetite for scrutinizing the tactics of the powerful food lobby, but the pressure to curb consumption of ultra-processed foods is growing.

More than 30 percent of young people aged 17 to 24 no longer qualify for US military service because of their weight. Diet-related ailments such as cardiovascular disease, cancer and diabetes soaked up 54% of the U.S. government's $383.6 billion in healthcare spending, which includes Medicare and Medicaid, in 2018.[6]

The American food system is not broken; it is functioning as designed—a system optimized for efficiency, not one optimized for resilience and nutrition. But our food system is killing us, and that happened long before Covid-19. It is bound to continue unless we take steps now to leverage food as medicine.[7]

Diet-related disease, which includes obesity, heart attack, strokes, cancer, and dementia, is the leading cause of early death in the UK. Driving it is a set of industrially processed products that are sold as food, known formally as ultra-processed food (UPF). Limiting the marketing of ultra-processed foods is essential. We need to learn the lessons from regulating the tobacco industry and stop predatory companies from selling this food to people. We need to end the conflict of interest among the food industry and politicians, doctors, and scientists.[8]

As noted in the *Wall Street Journal* on June 19, 2023, foods are stripped of nutrients and loaded with ingredients that contribute to disease. They're made to be addictive, too. An ultra-processed food is anything that's "wrapped in plastic and has at least one ingredient that you wouldn't usually find in a standard home kitchen."

Ultra-processed food is established as a metabolic disruptor acting to increase adiposity, reduce mitochondrial efficiency, drive insulin resistance, alter growth, and contribute to human morbidity and mortality. Chronic metabolic diseases (including type 2 diabetes, hypertension, dyslipidemia, cardiovascular disease, cancer, dementia, polycystic ovarian disease, and non-alcoholic fatty liver disease) are now rampant throughout both the developed and developing world.[9]

Ultra-processed foods (chips, candy, and chicken nuggets) make up 60% of the calories Americans consume, according to one study. Created by combining extracted parts from many different foods or synthetic ingredients, like preservatives, these Frankenstein foods contribute to poor health outcomes, such as insulin resistance, inflammation, and obesity.[10]

UNHEALTHY FOODS AREN'T JUST BAD FOR YOU; THEY MAY ALSO BE ADDICTIVE

The *New York Times* noted, " At the top of the list were pizza, chocolate, potato chips, cookies, ice cream, French fries and cheeseburgers. Like cigarettes and cocaine, their ingredients are derived from naturally occurring plants and foods that are stripped of components that slow their absorption, such as fiber, water and protein. Then their most pleasurable ingredients are refined and processed into products that are rapidly absorbed into the bloodstream, enhancing their ability to light up regions of the brain that regulate reward, emotion, and motivation".[11]

For males and females, sugar intake results in significant hormonal problems—and perhaps most shockingly, new evidence proves that sugar shrinks your hippocampus, which is your memory center. So, the next time you have a sugar craving, think about how it may literally shrink your brain cells! The human body never evolved to consume the levels of sugar in most diets today. Human physiology evolved on a diet containing very little sugar and virtually no refined carbohydrates. Ninety-three percent of Americans are metabolically unhealthy: they have high blood sugar, high cholesterol, high blood pressure, they're overweight, or they have had a heart attack or a stroke. This means, in effect, that a mere 6% of us are in good metabolic health. And Dr. Mark Hyman notes, "that's driven by our diet primarily."[12]

SUGAR IS DRIVING THE DIABETES AND DEPRESSION EPIDEMICS

Diabetes status, poor glycemic control, and longer diabetes duration remain associated with worse cognitive outcomes in persons evaluated at ages 66–90 years. In older adults with diabetes, maintaining glycemic control is an important avenue for mitigating cognitive impairments into older age.[13] Diabetes will be 'a defining disease of this century' as global cases are set to surpass one billion by 2050.[14]

SUGAR AND PROCESSED FOODS ARE LINKED TO MENTAL HEALTH, DEPRESSION, AND ALZHEIMER'S

High blood sugar can gradually damage the blood vessels in the brain. If the brain does not receive enough blood, brain cells can die, impacting a person's memory and thinking. Diabetes also increases a person's risk for stroke and heart disease, which can both heighten Alzheimer's risk. Elevated blood sugar may also cause inflammation in the brain, harming brain cells, and possibly contributing to Alzheimer's disease.[15]

A 2013 study found that insulin resistance and blood glucose levels —which are hallmarks of diabetes—are linked with a greater risk for developing neurodegenerative disorders like Alzheimer's. The research "offers more evidence that the brain is a target organ for damage by high blood sugar."

Chronically high blood sugar levels have also been linked to inflammation in the brain. And, as some research has suggested, neuroinflammation is one possible cause of depression. Research has also found that people who eat a standard American diet that is high in processed foods—which typically contain high amounts of saturated fat, sugar and salt—are at an increased risk for developing depression, compared to those who eat a whole foods diet that is lower in sugar, endocrinologist Dr. Medha Munshi told the *New York Times*.

For Alzheimer's, as with cancer—but also as with other conditions like heart disease and diabetes—much of the risk is related to behavioral and lifestyle factors. The consensus among scientists is that over one-third of all Alzheimer's cases could be prevented by improving our lifestyles. This includes increasing cardiovascular fitness, keeping our brains intellectually stimulated, and perhaps most of all, eating better.

"Eating better" means addressing the American ultra-processed diet. Ultra-processed is a technical term, and exists in a spectrum of food processing. Ultra-processed foods, by some measures, account for half of the American diet. The implications are clear. If, as a nation, we have become aware of the role of nutrition relative to cancer, it's urgent that we develop a corollary awareness of the role of nutrition and Alzheimer's. It's terrifying news because of the numbers we see ahead.[16] Eating packaged foods like cereal and frozen meals has been associated with anxiety, depression and cognitive decline. Seventy percent of the packaged foods sold in the United States are considered ultra-processed.[17] People who consume high amounts of ultra-processed foods report significantly more adverse mental health symptoms.[18]

This information is coming to the forefront at a time when Americans' self-reports of mental health are their worst in over two decades. More US adults—particularly those who are younger—are seeking help.[19] According to the CDC, one-third of US teen girls seriously considered attempting suicide in 2021. The number of teen girls who made a suicide plan also increased from 2019.[20]

Maybe it is time to start doing some real research and start to connect the dots between what we eat and the growing epidemic of poor mental health and depression?

THE LINK BETWEEN HIGHLY PROCESSED FOODS AND BRAIN HEALTH

Junk Food and the Brain: How Modern Diets Lacking in Micronutrients May Contribute to Angry Rhetoric.

We are being cheated of micronutrients (minerals and vitamins), particularly in those whose food choices are dominated by ultra-processed products.

To support brain metabolism, our brains require at least 30 micronutrients to ensure the production of neurotransmitters such as serotonin and dopamine, as well as breaking down and removing metabolic byproducts. Many studies of multi-nutrient treatments have found improved mood regulation and reduced irritability and explosive rage, including in placebo-controlled randomized trials of children with attention deficit hyperactivity disorder and mood dysregulation.

The evidence is clear: a well-nourished population is better able to withstand stress. Hidden brain hunger is one modifiable factor contributing to emotional outbursts, aggression, and even the loss of civility in public discourse.[21]

Excess consumption of refined sugars affects the human brain in ways similar to drugs like cocaine and may be even more addictive. That means sugar is just as habit-forming as narcotic drugs—and just as bad for us.

And did you know that long-term excess sugar consumption reduces dopamine levels and causes a reduction in the brain's dopamine receptors? When dopamine levels drop as a result of long-term consumption of sugar, the brain requires ever-higher levels of sugar consumption to reach the same reward levels and avoid mild states of depression. Drugs like cocaine, morphine and nicotine are addictive for the same reason—their effect on dopamine levels.[22]

One in five Americans today is living with a mental illness, according to the National Institutes of Mental Health. Depression, anxiety, schizophrenia, bipolar disorder, and autism are all more common now than they used to be. Energy shortfalls caused by mitochondrial dysfunction cause the brain to fail in predictable ways, and psychiatric symptoms or disorders are the result. People with obesity, diabetes, and other metabolic conditions are much, much more likely to develop mental illnesses such as depression, anxiety, and bipolar disorder.

Dr. Christian Palmer, MD is a neuroscientist and assistant professor of psychiatry at Harvard Medical School. In his new book, *Brain Energy*, Dr. Plummer describes how his clinical experience led him to explore the connection between metabolic dysfunction and mental disorder. By taking patients off of sugar, high carbohydrates, and processed foods, Dr. Palmer is getting much better results than prescribing pills and will soon be doing some blind placebo clinical trials to prove these results.

I will offer this observation: if you were to research or look at the charts for sugar and processed food consumption in the United States and compare those charts and trendlines to the increases in depression, suicide, ADHD, and Alzheimer's, the charts are scarily similar.

The proof is coming soon as Dr. Christian Plummer is setting up clinical trials to prove his thesis. Finally, we will have proof that sugar and processed foods, besides making you fat and sick, can also make you mentally ill.

I will close with this powerful quote by Dr. Lustig: "Sugar is the payload. Ultra-processed foods, the vehicle. That's the way to look at it. There's the atomic bomb, and there's the missile that delivers it."

SUGAR AFFECTS EYESIGHT

Findings by the NIH show an interaction between dietary carbohydrates, the gut microbiome, specific biochemical molecules, and Age-related Macular Degeneration (AMD) features. This work should lead to new approaches to understand, diagnose, and treat early AMD—perhaps before it affects vision. Already anticipated by human epidemiologic studies, the findings imply that we can optimize nutrition to prevent the progression of AMD.[23]

SUGAR LINKS TO CANCER

Increases Colon Cancer: A study by Harvard Medical School of 40,000 American women found those who ate the most foods with the highest glycemic index—a number that dictates how quickly sugar levels in the blood rise after eating it—had a three times higher risk of getting colon cancer than women who ate lesser amounts of these foods. Another study in 50,000 men found similar results.

Increases Pancreatic Cancer: A study in Sweden found that consuming added sugar increased the risk of pancreatic cancer by 69% over people who ate the least sugar.

Increases Prostate Cancer: An Italian study found that men whose diets were more likely to trigger an increase in blood sugar levels had a 57% higher risk of getting prostate cancer.

Increases Endometrial and Breast Cancer: The Iowa Women's Health Study examined 23,000 postmenopausal women. Researchers found that those who consumed a diet most likely to raise blood sugar levels experienced a 46% higher risk of getting endometrial cancer. For breast cancer the increase in cancer risk was a remarkable 135%.

Increase in *All* Cancers: After studying 1.3 million men and women in Korea for ten years, researchers found that those with the highest fasting glucose levels were more likely to develop cancer of all types.[24]

Sugar in fruit juice may raise risk of cancer: A study, carried out in France, was the first substantial piece of research to find a specific association between sugar and cancer. Fruit juices showed the same association with cancer as colas. "The main driver of the association seems to be sugar, so when we just look at the sugar content per 100ml, regular Coke or 100% orange juice, for instance, are quite the same."[25]

A BULLET-POINT SUMMARY OF HOW SUGAR DESTROYS OUR LIVES AND KILLS US SOFTLY

Nancy Appleton, PhD earned her BS in clinical nutrition from UCLA and her PhD in health services from Walden University. An avid researcher, Dr. Appleton is the best-selling author of *Stopping Inflamma-*

tion: Healthy Bones, and Lick the Sugar Habit. This is her truth about sugar checklist:

146 WAYS SUGAR RUINS YOUR HEALTH

by Nancy Appleton, ND, PhD in Nutrition

1. Sugar can suppress the immune system.
2. Sugar upsets the mineral relationships in the body.
3. Sugar can cause hyperactivity, anxiety, difficulty concentrating, and crankiness in children.
4. Sugar can produce a significant rise in triglycerides.
5. Sugar contributes to reduced defense against bacterial infection.
6. Sugar causes a loss of tissue elasticity and function; the more sugar you eat the more elasticity and function you lose.
7. Sugar reduces high-density lipoproteins.
8. Sugar leads to chromium deficiency.
9. Sugar leads to cancer of the breast, ovaries, prostrate, and rectum.
10. Sugar causes increased fasting levels of glucose.
11. Sugar causes copper deficiency.
12. Sugar interferes with absorption of calcium and magnesium.
13. Sugar can weaken eyesight.
14. Sugar raises the level of neurotransmitters: dopamine, serotonin, and norepinephrine.
15. Sugar can cause hypoglycemia.
16. Sugar can produce an acidic digestive tract.
17. Sugar can cause a rapid rise of adrenaline levels in children.
18. Sugar malabsorption is frequent in patients with functional bowel disease.
19. Sugar can cause premature aging.
20. Sugar can lead to alcoholism.
21. Sugar causes tooth decay.
22. Sugar contributes to obesity.

23. High intake of sugar increases the risk of Crohn's disease & ulcerative colitis.
24. Sugar can cause changes found in people with gastric or duodenal ulcers.
25. Sugar can cause arthritis.
26. Sugar can cause asthma.
27. Sugar greatly assists the uncontrolled growth of candida albicans (yeast infections).
28. Sugar can cause gallstones.
29. Sugar can cause heart disease.
30. Sugar can cause appendicitis.
31. Sugar can cause multiple sclerosis.
32. Sugar can cause hemorrhoids.
33. Sugar can cause varicose veins.
34. Sugar can elevate glucose and insulin responses in oral contraceptive users.
35. Sugar can lead to periodontal disease.
36. Sugar can contribute to osteoporosis.
37. Sugar contributes to saliva acidity.
38. Sugar can cause a decrease in insulin sensitivity.
39. Sugar can lower the amount of Vitamin E in the blood.
40. Sugar can decrease growth hormone.
41. Sugar can increase cholesterol.
42. Sugar can increase the systolic blood pressure.
43. Sugar can cause drowsiness and decreased activity in children.
44. High sugar intake increases advanced glycation end products (AGEs) (sugar that is bound non-enzymatically to protein).
45. Sugar can interfere with the absorption of protein.
46. Sugar causes food allergies.
47. Sugar contributes to diabetes.
48. Sugar can cause toxemia during pregnancy.
49. Sugar can contribute to eczema in children.
50. Sugar can cause cardiovascular disease.
51. Sugar can impair the structure of DNA.

52. Sugar can change the structure of protein.
53. Sugar can make our skin age by changing the structure of collagen.
54. Sugar can cause cataracts.
55. Sugar can cause emphysema.
56. Sugar can cause atherosclerosis.
57. Sugar can promote an elevation of low-density lipoproteins (LDL).
58. High sugar intake can impair the physiological homeostasis of many systems in the body.
59. Sugar lowers the enzymes' ability to function.
60. Sugar intake is higher in people with Parkinson's disease.
61. Sugar can permanently alter the way the proteins act in the body.
62. Sugar can increase the size of the liver by making the liver cells divide.
63. Sugar can increase the amount of liver fat.
64. Sugar can increase kidney size & produce pathological changes in the kidney.
65. Sugar can damage the pancreas.
66. Sugar can increase the body's fluid retention.
67. Sugar is enemy number one of the bowel movement.
68. Sugar can cause myopia (nearsightedness).
69. Sugar can compromise the lining of the capillaries.
70. Sugar can make the tendons more brittle.
71. Sugar can cause headaches, including migraine.
72. Sugar plays a role in pancreatic cancer in women.
73. Sugar can adversely affect schoolchildren's grades & cause learning disorders.
74. Sugar can cause an increase in delta, alpha, and theta brain waves.
75. Sugar can cause depression.
76. Sugar increases the risk of gastric cancer.
77. Sugar and cause dyspepsia (indigestion).
78. Sugar can increase your risk of getting gout.

79. Sugar can increase the levels of glucose in an oral glucose tolerance test over the ingestion of complex carbohydrates.
80. Sugar increases the insulin responses in humans consuming high-sugar diets compared to low-sugar diets.
81. A high refined-sugar diet reduces learning capacity.
82. Sugar can cause less effective functioning of two blood proteins, albumin, and lipoproteins, which may reduce the body's ability to handle fat and cholesterol.
83. Sugar can contribute to Alzheimer's disease.
84. Sugar can cause platelet adhesiveness.
85. Sugar can cause hormonal imbalance; some hormones become underactive, and others become overactive.
86. Sugar can lead to the formation of kidney stones.
87. Sugar can lead to the hypothalamus to become highly sensitive to a large variety of stimuli.
88. Sugar can lead to dizziness.
89. Diets high in sugar can cause free radicals and oxidative stress.
90. High-sucrose diets of subjects with peripheral vascular disease increases platelet adhesion.
91. A high-sugar diet can lead to biliary tract cancer.
92. Sugar feeds cancer.
93. High sugar consumption of pregnant adolescents is associated with a twofold increased risk for delivering a small-for-gestational-age (SGA) infant.
94. High sugar consumption can lead to a substantial decrease in gestation duration among adolescents.
95. Sugar slows food's travel time through the gastrointestinal tract.
96. Sugar increases the concentration of bile acids in stools and bacterial enzymes in the colon.
97. Sugar increases estradiol (the most potent form of naturally occurring estrogen) in men.
98. Sugar combines and destroys phosphatase, an enzyme, which makes the process of digestion more difficult.
99. Sugar can be a risk factor of gallbladder cancer.

100. Sugar is an addictive substance.
101. Sugar can be intoxicating, similar to alcohol.
102. Sugar can exacerbate PMS.
103. Sugar given to premature babies can affect the amount of carbon dioxide they produce.
104. Decrease in sugar intake can increase emotional stability.
105. The body changes sugar into two to five times more fat in the bloodstream than it does starch.
106. The rapid absorption of sugar promotes excessive food intake in obese subjects.
107. Sugar can worsen the symptoms of children with attention deficit hyperactivity disorder (ADHD).
108. Sugar adversely affects urinary electrolyte composition.
109. Sugar can slow down the ability of the adrenal glands to function.
110. Sugar has the potential of inducing abnormal metabolic processes in a normal healthy individual and promoting chronic degenerative diseases.
111. IVs (intravenous feedings) of sugar water can cut off oxygen to the brain.
112. High sucrose intake could be an important risk factor in lung cancer.
113. Sugar can increase the risk of polio.
114. High sugar intake can cause epileptic seizures.
115. Sugar causes high blood pressure in obese people.
116. In intensive care units, limiting sugar saves lives.
117. Sugar may induce cell death.
118. Sugar may impair the physiological homeostasis of many systems in living organisms.
119. In juvenile rehabilitation camps, when children were put on a low-sugar diet, there was a 44% drop in antisocial behavior.
120. Sugar can cause gastric cancer.
121. Sugar dehydrates newborns.
122. Sugar can cause gum disease.
123. Sugar increases the estradiol in young men.

124. Sugar can cause low birth weight babies.
125. Greater consumption of refined sugar is associated with a worse outcome of schizophrenia.
126. Sugar can raise homocysteine levels in the bloodstream.
127. Sweet food items increase the risk of breast cancer.
128. Sugar is a risk factor in cancer of the small intestine.
129. Sugar may cause laryngeal cancer.
130. Sugar induces salt and water retention.
131. Sugar may contribute to mild memory loss.
132. As sugar increases in the diet of ten year olds, there is a linear decrease in the intake of many essential nutrients.
133. Sugar can increase the total amount of food consumed.
134. Exposing a newborn to sugar results in a heightened preference for sucrose relative to water at six months and two years of age.
135. Sugar causes constipation.
136. Sugar can cause liver tumors.
137. Sugar can cause brain decay in prediabetic and diabetic women.
138. Sugar can increase the risk of stomach cancer.
139. Sugar causes metabolic syndrome.
140. Sugar ingestion by pregnant women increases neural tube defects in embryos.
141. Sugar can be a factor in asthma.
142. The higher the sugar consumption, the higher the chances of getting irritable bowel syndrome.
143. Sugar could affect central reward systems.
144. Sugar can cause cancer of the rectum.
145. Sugar can cause endometrial cancer.
146. Sugar can cause renal (kidney) cell carcinoma.

The war on drugs has failed because we keep going after the source and distribution rather than the education of the consumer. We are losing the war on sugar as its advocates (those making money from its sale, distribution, use and treatment of the problems) are a far stronger and more entrenched adversary, dwarfing the power and influence of the drug cartels. At this time our only chance is to educate our sugar addicts by whatever means possible.

Hopefully, by reading this chapter you have somehow connected the dots that sugar and its evil twin, processed food, are bad for your health, and will lead to the last quarter of your life being your worst quarter. They will cause you to waste lots of time and money on visiting doctors and hospitals, suffer needlessly, and have an unnecessary premature death. However, the good news is, the human body is amazing in its ability to cure itself, if given the chance.

CHAPTER 11
THE ANTI-SUGAR GODFATHERS

I used *Godfather in the chapter title* to catch your attention as many believe the original movie was one of the top movies of all time. So, yes, it is an attention getter. But the real reasons are threefold. The first is to remind us how powerful the entrenched money interests (who couldn't care less about our good health and are more concerned about their pocketbooks and placating shareholders) are. The second reason is to remind us how we must be concerned that all of what we are being told by the news media, medical establishments, governments, and other sources of news and information may not be true. Thirdly, at the end of this book, just like Don Corleone, if you wish to live, I will make you an offer that you cannot refuse.

So, with this in mind please read on.

SKEPTICS AND CONSPIRACY THEORISTS ARE RIGHT SOMETIMES

Throughout history, there have been numerous instances where famous individuals made significant discoveries but faced skepticism and ridicule before their ideas were accepted.

Here are a few examples:

Nicolaus Copernicus (1473-1543): Copernicus proposed the heliocentric model of the solar system, stating that the Earth revolves around the sun. This contradicted the prevailing geocentric model, which placed the earth at the center of the universe. Copernicus faced opposition from the church and many scholars of his time.

Galileo Galilei (1564-1642): Galileo's observations using a telescope supported Copernicus's heliocentric model. He discovered the four largest moons of Jupiter, observed the phases of Venus, and identified sunspots. His ideas were met with resistance from the Catholic church, and he was accused of heresy.

Gregor Mendel (1822-1884): Mendel, an Augustinian monk, conducted experiments with pea plants and formulated the laws of inheritance. However, his work was largely overlooked and not widely accepted during his lifetime. It wasn't until years after his death that his discoveries were recognized as the foundation of modern genetics.

Ignaz Semmelweis (1818-1865): Semmelweis, a Hungarian physician, advocated for handwashing to prevent the spread of infectious diseases in hospitals. His ideas were met with ridicule by his colleagues, and he faced significant opposition. His efforts to improve hygiene practices were not widely accepted until long after his death.

Rosalind Franklin (1920-1958): Franklin was a British chemist and X-ray crystallographer who played a crucial role in discovering the structure of DNA. Her work produced vital evidence for the double-helix structure, but she faced significant challenges and was not given due credit during her lifetime.

These individuals faced skepticism and ridicule, but their groundbreaking discoveries eventually gained recognition and significantly contributed to the advancement of science.

You can add John Yudkin to this list.

JOHN YUDKIN: THE ORIGINAL ANTI-SUGAR GODFATHER

John Yudkin was a British physiologist and nutritionist who is best known for his research on the relationship between sugar consumption and health. He was born on August 8, 1910 and passed away on July 12, 1995. Yudkin served as the chair of nutrition at Queen Elizabeth College, University of London, and was a prominent figure in the field of nutrition science during his time.

Yudkin gained significant attention and faced controversy for his views on the role of sugar in the development of various health conditions, particularly heart disease and obesity. In 1972, he published a book titled *Pure, White, and Deadly,* in which he argued that excessive consumption of sugar, specifically refined sugar and high-fructose corn syrup, contributed to a range of health problems. He suggested that sugar, rather than dietary fat, was the primary cause of obesity and related diseases. This well-written and factual book sounded the alarm that sugar—and not fat—was the greatest danger to our health and the cause of obesity, coronary disease, and related diseases.

However, Yudkin's views were met with significant criticism and skepticism from other researchers, as well as industries that benefited from the consumption of sugar. At the time, the prevailing belief in nutrition science focused more on the role of dietary fat in health issues, such as heart disease. Yudkin's theories were largely dismissed and ridiculed, and he faced challenges in gaining acceptance for his research.

In his book he noted that "If only a small fraction of what we know about the effects of sugar were to be revealed in relation to any other material used as a food additive, that material would promptly be banned." The book did well, but Yudkin paid a high price for it. Prominent nutritionists combined with the food industry worked to destroy his reputation, and his career never recovered. He died, in 1995, a disappointed, largely forgotten man.

When Yudkin was conducting his research into the effects of sugar in the 1960s, a new nutritional orthodoxy was in the process of asserting itself. Its central tenet was that a healthy diet is a low-fat diet. Yudkin led a diminishing band of dissenters who believed that sugar, not fat, was the more likely cause of maladies such as obesity, heart disease, and diabetes. But by the time he wrote his book, the commanding heights of the field had been seized by proponents of the fat hypothesis.

The leader of the anti-fat movement was a nutritionist at the University of Minnesota, Ancel Keys. Ancel Keys was brilliant, charismatic, and combative. He was intensely aware that Yudkin's sugar hypothesis posed an alternative to his own. If Yudkin published a paper, Keys would excoriate it, and him. He called Yudkin's theory "a mountain of nonsense," and accused him of issuing "propaganda" for the meat and dairy industries. Yudkin never responded in kind. He was a mild-mannered man, unskilled in the art of political combat. The British Sugar Bureau dismissed Yudkin's claims about sugar as "emotional assertions," and the World Sugar Research Organization called his book "science fiction."

Throughout the 1960s, Keys accumulated institutional power. He secured places for himself and his allies on the boards of the most influential bodies in American healthcare, including the American Heart Association and the National Institutes of Health.

And Keys held a trump card. From 1958 to 1964, he and his fellow researchers gathered data on the diets, lifestyles, and health of 12,770 middle-aged men, in Italy, Greece, Yugoslavia, Finland, Netherlands, Japan, and the United States. *The Seven Countries Study* was finally published as a 211-page monograph in 1970. It showed a correlation between intake of saturated fats and deaths from heart disease, just as Keys had predicted.

However, the study was of shaky construction. There was no objective basis for the countries chosen by Keys. After all, why choose seven nations in Europe and leave out France and Germany? Maybe because the French and Germans had relatively low rates of heart disease, despite living on a diet rich in saturated fats, thus contradicting Key's assertions?

In fact, one can look at many tribes and cultures around the world and see many contradicting facts to *The Seven Countries Study*. Consider the following examples:

Inuit (Eskimos): The traditional diet of the Inuit people in the Arctic region consists mainly of fish, marine mammals, and other animal products. Their diet is naturally high in fat, particularly omega-3 fatty acids from fish. Despite consuming a diet rich in saturated fats, the Inuit historically had low rates of heart disease. However, it's worth noting that recent changes in their dietary patterns due to increased consumption of processed and Westernized foods have led to a rise in heart disease and other health issues.

Maasai: The Maasai people of East Africa traditionally rely on a diet that includes meat, milk, and blood from their livestock, such as cattle. Their diet is high in animal fats, yet heart disease was virtually nonexistent among the Maasai until the introduction of a more Westernized diet.

Mediterranean populations: While not typically characterized as high-fat diets, Mediterranean diets are moderate in total fat but include higher proportions of healthy fats, such as olive oil, nuts, and fish. Populations in Mediterranean countries, such as Greece, Italy, and Spain, have historically demonstrated lower rates of heart disease despite consuming relatively high-fat diets. This may be attributed to the overall dietary pattern, which includes abundant fruits, vegetables, whole grains, and a moderate intake of red wine.

Tokelau: The Tokelauan people, inhabitants of the South Pacific, traditionally consume a diet rich in coconut products, which are high in saturated fat. Despite their high-fat diet, Tokelauans had low rates of heart disease until the introduction of processed foods and sugar in their diets, leading to an increase in heart disease rates.

But this and other evidence was ignored. John Yudkin's scientific reputation had been all but sunk. He found himself uninvited from international conferences on nutrition. Research journals refused his papers. He was talked about by fellow scientists as an eccentric, a lone obsessive. Eventually, he became an uncertain story. Professor John Yudkin retired from his post at Queen Elizabeth College in 1971, to write *Pure, White and Deadly*. However, a final slap in the face was the College reneged on its agreement to give him a space for future writings and research.

In recent years, there has been renewed interest in Yudkin's work as emerging research has supported many of his findings regarding the potential negative health effects of excessive sugar consumption. His contributions to the understanding of the relationship between sugar and health have been recognized posthumously, and he is considered a pioneer in the field of nutrition science.

DR. ROBERT H. LUSTIG: THE NEW ANTI-SUGAR GODFATHER

Enter stage left, the new godfather of the anti-sugar movement, Dr. Robert Lustig. Dr Lustig is an internationally renowned pediatric endocrinologist and now attorney, who has spent 15+ years treating childhood obesity and studying the effects of sugar on the central nervous system, metabolism and chronic disease. He is the *New York Times* bestselling author of *Fat Chance, Hacking of the American Mind*, and *Metabolical*. Additionally, his 2009 YouTube video, "Sugar: The Bitter Truth" lecture to some graduate students at the University of California has now received more than 25 million views, probably the most of any graduate school lecture in history.

In 2008 Dr. Lustig gave a talk at the Australasian Association of Clinical Biochemists and a doctor said, "surely you must have read Yudkin." Dr. Lustig had not, and obtained a copy of *Pure, White and Deadly*. Lustig realized Yudkin's work pre-dated his by a whopping 36 years. Later when Lustig was asked why he was the first major researcher in years to focus on the dangers of sugar, he answered: "John Yudkin. They took him down so severely—so severely—that nobody wanted to attempt it on their own."

Dr. Lustig wrote a very moving introduction to the 2012 edition of *Pure, White and Deadly*. It was a tribute to the unappreciated and forgotten man John Yudkin. Lustig notes, "Sadly, interpretation of medical science is frequently influenced by the dark forces of industry, out to make a killing." He cites Big Tobacco as one major example. Lustig goes on to say that John Yudkin's book "was, is and remains, a prophecy...He preached in the wilderness and nobody listened." Dr. Lustig covers the background of some of the flawed beliefs of that time such as Ancel Keys's incorrect "fat is bad " hypothesis, which included the claims that LDL was a major cause of heart attacks and fat can raise LDL.

In his closing, Dr. Lustig writes that Yudkin correctly fingered the sugar and food industries as being villains. He states "I am proud to be a Yudkin disciple, ... Every scientist stands on the shoulders of giants. For a man of relatively diminutive stature and build, Dr. John Yudkin was indeed a giant."

From all my research, I can say without any doubt that Dr. Robert Lustig is indeed the new truth-telling, informed, factual, and dedicated anti-sugar prophet. He has zeroed in on the perils of sugar consumption and processed foods and is leading the charge (hence the new law degree) to right the world's ship of poor health and to carry on John Yudkin's truth-telling anti-sugar torch.

CHAPTER 12
THE COCAINE
CONNECTION

T he majority of people in this world have a healthy disrespect for cocaine (except for the addicts, of course). Conversely, the majority of people in this world have a healthy love of sugar. As noted previously, sugar products are their feel good, taste good comfort foods.

This is the reason I have written this chapter. I want to perhaps shock you into understanding not only sugar's nature but its similarity to something the majority of us despise and will never consume.

Since you avoid cocaine, should you not avoid sugar if it is just as bad for you?

In the process of trying to understand the incredible appeal and addiction to sugar, I stumbled onto an uncanny comparison of cocaine to sugar.

I would like to back up a bit. I have written this chapter with the voice of experience. To this day I can remember the article in *Playboy* in the mid 70s extolling the virtues of cocaine and how it was a harmless, hedonistic drug that was starting to hit the discos, bars, parties, and private jets of the rich and famous. So, I experimented with it for several years and soon discovered it is what I will call a zero-sum drug with diminishing returns.

From my own personal experience experimenting with cocaine, I recall the feeling of the diminishing highs and the later lows as you crash the next day. The negative energy and the low-lows over time more than offset the diminished highs, and that was enough for me to walk away. This experience, combined with accurate news from the medical community, the government and the main street media, it was an easy decision to quit it for good.

But I never understood the highs and lows of sugar. They were not as obvious for me as I was not that big of a sugar consumer. But for some sugar users, these can be more pronounced.

Cocaine users (perhaps about 35 million in the US from a recent national survey on drug abuse), you might find this chapter interesting. For sugar users (99% of the people reading this book) who fear using cocaine for all the obvious reasons, hopefully this will be a wakeup call and an additional clue that sugar is bad for your health.

My hope is that for those of you who are terrified of cocaine, after looking at this chart below, you will see that sugar is just as insidious and this might help you give up the sugar drug just like you would the cocaine drug.

FEATURES	COCAINE	SUGAR
White powder or crystalline form	✓	✓
Stimulates dopamine pleasure centers	✓	✓
Lead to poor health and even death over long-term usage	✓	✓
Is used socially	✓	✓
Comes from a plant	✓	✓
Can be smoked	✓	✓ (sugar is added to tobacco)
Can be chewed	✓ (leaf)	✓ (tobacco and gum)
Is highly addictive	✓	✓
Withdrawal problems	✓	✓
The high diminishes over time requiring more of the drug to get the same effect	✓	✓
Is a processed plant	✓	✓
Was in the original formula for Coca Cola	✓	✓
Negatively effects normal sleep	✓	✓
Can cause weight loss	✓	✗
Is illegal	✓	✗
Is expensive in Western countries	✓	✗

From this chart you can see that cocaine is better in one category, and that is at least you can lose some weight. In the future, if it gets legalized, then it will be the same in every category as sugar except for the weight loss. I know for some, it is hard to believe that sugar is such a close relative to cocaine, but the facts speak for themselves.

Poor Pablo Escobar, who in 1987, was listed by *Forbes* as one of the ten richest men in the world. If Pablo had been growing and distributing sugar instead, with his great marketing acumen, he would probably be alive today and richer than Elon Musk and Jeff Bezos. Unfortunately for him, he chose the wrong drug.

In closing I did leave off one comparison: cocaine can kill you quicker, whereas sugar kills you softly, sweetly, and slowly.

CHAPTER 13
WOMEN'S LOVE AFFAIR WITH SUGAR

Women's love affair with sugar is a complex and multifaceted issue, and there are several reasons why women may find themselves craving sweet foods.

First, sugar activates the reward centers in the brain, leading to the release of feel-good chemicals such as dopamine. This can create a pleasurable sensation that reinforces the desire for more sugar. Women may be particularly vulnerable to this effect due to hormonal fluctuations throughout the menstrual cycle that can impact mood and cravings.

Second, women may use sugar as a coping mechanism for stress or negative emotions. Eating sweet foods can provide a temporary distraction from unpleasant feelings and can help to boost mood and energy levels. Men, on the other hand, may head to the bar to drown their sorrows.

Third, social and cultural factors may also play a role in women's love affair with sugar. Sweet foods are often associated with comfort, celebration, and indulgence, and can be a way to bond with others or mark special occasions.

This is probably my most difficult chapter to write because if taken the wrong way, it may ruffle some feathers. In this day of political correctness, wokeness, and the me-too movement, then I probably should tread lightly about suggesting that women are our biggest sugar consumption violators.

TRADITIONALLY, WOMEN ARE OUR GATEKEEPERS

I am going to take a chance and say what needs to be said, to wake up our gatekeepers, as women tend to be the biggest influence on what children, husbands, and boyfriends eat. If our gatekeepers have a love affair with sugar, then bad things will happen to our children.

Thinking back to my birth on Mar 10, 1944, I was pretty lucky to have made it out OK. During her pregnancy, my mom smoked cigarettes (doctors were recommending them at that time) and she drank her martinis (the negative link to alcohol and pregnancy had not yet been established). Fortunately, she was not doing drugs and, most fortunately, she was eating real food. She was not eating pizza, fast food, or processed foods, but instead was mainly eating real food, which was the norm in the 1940s. Also, I caught a bit of a break in that the processed food, fast food, and Big Pill industries were emerging around me as I was growing up. Thus, I survived to tell this story.

For today's babies it is a different story. Responsible pregnant moms today are not drinking booze, not taking drugs and not smoking. Such great moms they are, but unfortunately, they are uninformed and highly addicted moms. During pregnancy this is their main food craving list:

- Ice cream
- Chocolate
- Pickles
- Red Meat
- Peanut butter
- Potato chips
- Spicy foods
- Sweets (chocolate, candy)
- Savory high-calorie carbohydrates (pizza, chips)
- Savory high-calorie dairy (cheese, sour cream, yogurt with sugar added)

- Carbohydrates (pretzels, cereal, pasta, rice)
- Fast food (Chinese, Mexican, burgers, pizza, sandwiches)
- Cold foods (ice pops, slushies)
- Sweet high-calorie dairy (ice cream, milkshakes, sundaes).

Do you see any pattern here? The vast majority of this food intake is high in sugar and heavily carb-loaded. Moms-to-be are loading up on the sugar and processed foods, and this is getting dumped into the placenta. Hence the results that Dr. Lustig and doctors across the US, and the world, are now seeing: babies being born obese, pre-diabetic and addicted to sugar, right out of the womb.

WHAT IS THE FOURTH GENERATION OF SUGAR ADDICTS GOING TO LOOK LIKE?

Research shows women are more likely than men to have a strong hankering for something sweet. According to a study published in *Appetite*, 97% of women and 68% of men who took part in a survey admitted to food cravings. Men and women tend to crave different kinds of foods. Several studies have shown that men report more craving for savory foods (e.g., meat, fish, eggs), whereas women report more craving for sweet foods (e.g., chocolate, pastries, ice cream). Further, men may crave different types of sweets than women do (e.g., sugar-sweetened beverages, but not chocolate). Consistently, a few studies have shown that more than 92% of those who experience strong cravings for chocolate are female.[1]

There is a widespread belief that women have a particular affinity for sugar, and this has been a topic of interest for researchers and scientists. However, it's important to note that not all women have a love affair with sugar, and there are many factors that can influence an individual's preference for sweet foods.

As previously noted, women may be more likely to crave sugary foods due to hormonal fluctuations. For example, during the menstrual cycle, estrogen and progesterone levels fluctuate, which can affect insulin sensitivity and increase the desire for sweet foods. Additionally, stress and anxiety can trigger cravings for sugar, and women may be more susceptible to these emotions due to societal pressures and expectations.

Also, cultural and social factors play a role in women's love affair with sugar. Many women are raised with the idea that sweets are a reward or a source of comfort, and they may associate them with positive experiences or emotions. Furthermore, women may be more likely to engage in emotional eating, which can involve turning to sugary foods as a way of coping with stress or negative emotions.

Our women have been marketed to and brainwashed with the idea that sweets = comfort food. That sugar gives them energy, comfort, makes them happy, increases serotonin (a lie), and that they deserve it as they suffer through the rough patches of their pregnancies. With this in mind and considering that even pre-pregnancy, most women are already sugar-addicted, the pregnancy simply delivers the hammer blow, in terms of increased sugar consumption.

We know from previous chapters that sugar is addictive, and this increases over time like any drug. The only way to beat it is to quit. The good news being that once you do so, the cravings go away.

My mission is to win our gatekeepers over and wean them off of sugar so they, their children, and their families will not suffer from sugar addiction and all of the unhealthy issues that it so drives.

Let's start with dinner. Think of the last time as a couple (husband and wife, lovers, friends, etc.) that you dined with other couples at a nice restaurant. You all have had a nice meal and after finishing, the waiter has cleaned the dishes and spruced up the table. What does the waiter say next?

¨WOULD YOU LIKE COFFEE OR DESSERT?¨

Now try to recall this picture, or better yet, go try it out at your next dinner out with couples. I want you to watch the eyes of the women at the table when the waiter mentions dessert. You will see a rise, a spark, as the pleasure hormone, dopamine, is released. Watch their eyes and then listen to what comes next. The women will nudge their male partner with their elbow and say, ¨Oh, that sounds nice. Why don't we share a dessert?¨ The male partner has nowhere to go but to agree to getting roped into having some sugar-infused dessert after such a great meal. He also is probably thinking he would rather have an after-dinner drink or perhaps a cigar. But the die is cast and there is no escaping driving up their insulin levels after the meal and stressing out their livers.

Another anecdote that I vividly recall was my post-skin-cancer surgery visit with my dermatologist in Medellin, Colombia. My dermatologist was also one of the few surgeons who could perform such a surgery so close to my eye, on the side of my nose. She was recommended to me by my dentist and happens to be his wife. Besides being a great doctor, she is also beautiful and in her early 40s. During my follow-up post-op visit, we were talking about a number of things and she mentioned that she was pre-diabetic. I, of course, immediately said to her, "you have to quit sugar." I will never forget the look in her eyes. It was almost as if I had stabbed her in the heart. She was having none of this and let me know it immediately so I dropped the subject.

Fast-forward a year and I am having a dental session with her husband and I was making real headway with him, as I have with a number of medical professionals, to educate them about the perils of sugar and all of the things that convert into sugar. He had gone from mildly interested in my rantings to becoming convinced that I was on to something. He was impressed that for the first time in about 70 years I had stopped developing cavities and I had no more plaque. He saw my new health and energy and that I looked better in my mid 70s than I had in my 60s. He not only got on board with the detoxing, quitting sugar, and eating real food, but he also became an advocate. He was studying the latest real research on sugar and processed foods like I was. In fact, he had moved on to anti-aging protocols.

Of course, I had to ask how things were at home with his sugar-loving spouse (my dermatologist) and, unfortunately, he said, there were arguments. She was enjoying her M&M's, Reese's Peanut Butter Cups, and sweets as these were her comfort food after a long, stressful day. She was not setting an example for their sons as he was trying to do, to extol the perils of sugar consumption. I am not sure how this will play out long term, and I hope my legacy will be saving lives and not destroying marriages. My point is that women love their sugar and it is a challenge to convert them, more so than men.

Offer a man and a woman a choice of a chocolate bar vs. a beer, hamburger, steak, beef jerky, etc. and you can see what the issue is. So, what are some motivations that we can offer to women?

Women want to look beautiful, but they often gain weight and lose the figures of their teens and twenties, due to sugar and processed-food consumption. Their skin is important, so as blemishes, spots, and wrinkles start to appear, they cover those with makeup. I wonder if they would be motivated to stop eating sugar if they knew that it is bad for their skin. Remember from the earlier science section, sugar has both browning and aging effects on skin that increase over time.

Just for the heck of it, I decided to put the sentence, "Is sugar bad for your skin" into the Internet's hottest website, ChatGBT. Here was the bot's answer:

> Eating too much sugar can contribute to the development of acne and other skin conditions. High blood sugar levels can lead to inflammation, which can make acne worse. Additionally, a diet high in sugar can cause wrinkles and age spots by breaking down collagen and elastin in the skin. To keep skin healthy, it is best to limit your intake of sugary foods and drinks.

Maybe I should hire the bot to promote my book?

I have experienced firsthand how my skin has improved since I quit sugar. I believe it would be the same for any man or woman. What is more beautiful than nice, natural makeup-free skin on a toned female body?

You may have noticed I slipped in the word toned, so now we are on to the next step to possibly upsetting some readers, but here goes. Remember I am hiding out in Colombia, so read on, but no retributions, please.

I have been going to the gym for weight training and cardio since 1995. I have to confess at age 55 I was fortunate to have dated a beautiful bodybuilder while living in Naples Florida. She lived in Ft. Lauderdale, but I did not mind the drive and I was fully motivated to take up weight lifting if it would offer me any chance of winning her heart. She even gave me some free weight training lessons. Fairly soon afterwards it appeared my charms were not enough to woo her, so she left me for another, but she also left me with a legacy of continuing to stay with the weight lifting. I have been doing it for 27 years, and continue today at age 79. Looking back, this is one of the reasons that I am still alive and was partly a reason I survived my metabolic syndrome up to the time I quit sugar.

I digress as I want to talk about my current time at the gym. Do you know what has been mostly missing at my gyms? Women my age. The prevailing wisdom might say weight lifting— and perhaps many outdoor sports —are more of a man's domain. There may be other reasons or notions why older women reduce high intensive exercise. But I have my own ideas and they have to do with sugar.

Remember previous information that the fructose in sugar reduces the production of ADP, our energy driver, and hence with lower energy we feel less and less like working out. Combine this with being overweight and skin that requires a lot of makeup, do you really believe a woman wants to go and workout at a gym, or anywhere else for that matter. The cycle continues every year: less energy, more weight, worse skin, and throw in a little depression and/or pill taking, and you have the perfect prescription for non-exercise.

Now the Big Three (eating real food, exercise, and sleep) are out the window (when the first two are not working, a good night's sleep is almost impossible). This is such a shame because in my opinion, nothing is more beautiful than a mature woman with beautiful skin and a great body; combined with wisdom and grace, the younger girls would not have a chance. I say this in all respect. I know that looks are not everything, but if they were not important, why would women be spending so much money on clothes, makeup, fashion, getting their hair done, Botox, plastic surgery, pills, lipo, etc.? The smartest, most important, and least expensive first step should be quitting sugar.

With sugar gone, the weight comes down and the energy goes up and bingo, we are on our way with a new outlook and a new body, a new glow, and a new confidence that will start attracting the opposite sex. Do you think Elizabeth Hurley, Michelle Pfeiffer, Kylie Minogue, Iman, Sophia Loren, Courtney Cox, Halle Berry, Sharon Stone, Selma Hayek, etc. eat a lot of sugar and processed foods? I bet if you check what they eat, they are not big sugar consumers, and they certainly are not overweight.

Women do most of the grocery shopping. They feed the kids but they are the ones typically giving the kids sweets and desserts. They influence what their husbands, boyfriends, or girlfriends will be eating and, in many cases, are cooking for them. They expect their chocolates on Valentine's Day. When they are out with the girls, they love to order desserts. Women tend to be dieting more than men. They use makeup to make their skin look better.

What most women do not do is quit sugar and processed foods. If they did, they could lose whatever weight they wished. Their skin would improve dramatically. They would have more energy. Varicose veins would be reduced, if not eliminated. They would feel more like exercising. If they applied the same regimen to their children, the children would be both healthier and better behaved. Women would be more attractive to their husbands, other men, or girlfriends, if that is the case. And there is evidence that sex lives for both men and women are improved when eating properly, exercising, and sleeping are optimized.

In conclusion, it is critical to get our gatekeepers on board to protect the children, to whip the guys into shape, and to attain the goal of having the last half of their lives engaged in living and loving in a healthy manner reminiscent of their youths.

CHAPTER 14
KILLING OUR KIDS

"Killing Our Kids" is, without a doubt, the most disturbing and important chapter to write. I purposely placed it after "Women's Love Affair with Sugar." Our children need informed, disciplined guidance. Moms are the key.

We should all be shocked and in a state of alarm when considering that in the 250 years of the United States of America, that today's generation of children *will not outlive their parents.*

This is unprecedented!

Previously I noted that today's babies are being born pre-diabetic, obese, and addicted to sugar right out of the womb. We laid the blame on the unhealthy sugar-laden and processed food diets of pregnant mothers. These moms are most likely unknowingly putting their babies at a big disadvantage at the very beginning of their child's lives. These toddlers, once addicted to sugar, fall lockstep into the sugar-infused and processed-food diets of their parents.

You may recall that Dr. Robert Lustig was initially a pediatric physician treating children with all sorts of maladies including diabetes; pre-diabetes; obesity; cardiovascular disease; asthma; all types of food allergies; gastrointestinal issues; skin issues like eczema, dermatitis, and acne; attention deficit hyperactivity disorder (ADHD); autism; and mental health conditions like anxiety disorders, depression, and behavioral disorders. Over time, and contrary to his medical training of prescribing pills for everything (thank you, Big Pharma), Dr. Lustig discovered the linkage to many of these maladies to sugar. Without a doubt, his endocrinology background facilitated his ability to connect the dots to sugar.

Dr. Lustig has personally witnessed over the past three decades that childhood obesity rates have tripled in the US, and today the country has some of the highest obesity rates in the world: one out of three children are overweight or obese.

We know that the main culprit for this rise in childhood obesity rates is *sugar*! Studies have revealed that 85% of infants and toddlers consume added sugar every single day.

 Nutritional biochemical or chemical injury is so much more enhanced early in life, in childhood, during pregnancy, and before the age of ten years old. There is a strong relationship between processed food and commercial baked goods and emotional injury to the brain increasing risk of later life, depression and anxiety. And also reducing intellectual success, scholastic and economic success. Parents really are the drug enablers white sugar is a drug. So, the celebration of birthdays and Halloween and school events and taking kids to feeding kids fast foods and sugar products is really the same thing as giving your kids cigarettes, sharing cocaine with them, and giving them whiskey.

DR. JOEL FUHRMAN

Very strong but truthful words indeed!

The May 2023 Sugar Free Kids Summit highlighted that the hidden dangers of sugar that are putting children's health at risk seem to be growing. Some of these hidden dangers include the following:

- Brain and developmental disorders
- Fatty liver disease
- Type 2 diabetes

- Type 1 diabetes
- Obesity
- Hyperactivity disorders
- Impaired cognitive function
- Inflammatory diseases like asthma
- Heart disease

As a baby boomer myself, and speaking with many other boomers, as children we did not see kids having these types of problems. Kids with ADHD taking Ritalin, never. Overweight kids, rare. Bad skin not so often. Diabetics, even rarer. Food allergies seemed far-fetched as we ate everything (unfortunately, also sugar, as we were the first generation of sugar addicts). The point is that the maladies of youth have gotten progressively worse with each generation and is now culminating with the current calamity of our kids not outliving their parents, in spite of having the greatest advancements in medicine in the history of mankind available today.

As our children grow up, what are they exposed to in their diets and eating regimens? Think about the traditions from the past 100 years that are now ensconced in their daily lives.

- Telling your children to eat all their dinner or they will not get a dessert.
- **Halloween** is a great time to get free bags full of candy and sweets (I remember trick-or-treating and being upset if a neighbor gave me an apple instead of a candy bar).
- On **Valentine's Day,** you can poison your sweetie pie with sugar-infused chocolates.
- If your wife or girlfriend is mad at you, send her a box of **chocolates**.
- If your kids are misbehaving or acting up, give them some **candy or ice cream** to distract them and calm them down (at least until the sugar high subsides).
- Parents want to talk to each other or with friends, so keep the kids at bay by giving them sweets so they will not bother you.

- Candy canes, gingerbread houses, cookies, and chocolate treats are traditional at **Christmas** time.
- The star event of all kids' **birthday parties** is not the opening of the presents, but rather the chowing down on cake, cupcakes and ice cream.
- **Easter eggs** (which are often made of chocolate or candy) and Easter egg hunts (where children search for hidden eggs filled with sweets) are beloved.
- **Diwali,** also known as the Festival of Lights, is a major Hindu festival celebrated in India and other parts of the world where sweets and desserts play a significant role.
- **Hanukkah** is a Jewish holiday where people light the menorah, play dreidel games, and enjoy traditional foods like sufganiyot (jelly-filled doughnuts) and gelt (chocolate coins).
- **Día de los Muertos** is a Mexican holiday with sugar skulls (calaveras de azúcar), and intricately decorated candy skulls are a significant part of the festivities.
- For **Mother's Day**, if you can´t take mom out to lunch, send her a box of chocolates.
- I'm not sure how it is today in the US, but last century many doctors' and **dentists' offices had jars of lollipops** for the kids to keep them distracted or happy.
- In Colombia it is traditional for restaurants to leave some candies or sweets with your bill at a restaurant.

These are just some of the traditions recently ingrained into many cultures and especially targeted to women and children. Some are indirectly targeted to men as they often wish to please a woman.

Now combine the above with the marketing of sugar-laced foods by Big Food. Keep in mind the dastardly marketing that Big Tobacco used to direct at kids in the last century. Now fast-forward to the 20th century where Big Tobacco is a major investor or owner in many of the largest processed-food companies. We can see some Big Tobacco's influence in creating alluring marketing campaigns aimed at kids to get them addicted early. Consider some of the following with their catchy ads shown during kids' TV shows:

- Fruit Loops
- Lucky Charms
- Cinnamon Toast Crunch
- Sugar Frosted Flakes – what kid can resist that friendly, cuddly Tony the Tiger?
- Cocoa Puffs
- Apple Jacks
- Honey Nut Cheerios
- Reese's Puffs
- Trix
- Cap'n Crunch

The above is just a list of popular cereals. The lists are much longer for other sugar-infused snacks, such as the following:

- Bubble gum (Double Bubble and Hubba Bubba)
- Chocolate bars like Hershey's Milk Chocolate, Kit Kat, Snickers, Milky Way, Reese's Peanut Butter Cups, and Twix
- Gummy bears, gummy worms, and other gummy candies by brands like Haribo, Trolli, and Albanese
- Candy such as Skittles, M&M's, Starburst, Sour Patch Kids, and Jolly Ranchers
- Soft drinks and sugared beverages such as Coca Cola, Sprite, Fanta, Dr. Pepper, Mountain Dew, Root Beer, lemonade, fruit juices, milk shakes, malts, Red Bull, fruit punch, slushies, etc.
- Other sugary favorites like all types of cookies, Oreos, marshmallows, popsicles, ice cream bars, donuts, cereal, granola bars, chocolate-covered snacks, etc.

What are parents, especially the mothers, doing to keep this garbage out of the mouths of their children? I suspect not much, as many moms and dads are indulging themselves. Our moms need to be the first line of defense in feeding children real food and creating healthy eating habits. Currently, we are losing this battle.

We all need to get on board and reverse this poisonous onslaught upon our kids. Some parents may be surprised to find out that if you inform your children of the truth and get them educated and trained early, they will become strong converts. Kids are not stupid. They are just disadvantaged with uninformed or lazy parents (or both). I have seen young kids who, once they understand about the perils of sugar and start eating real food, become incredible advocates for healthy eating and then have a positive influence on their peers.

But it all starts with the moms getting educated and on board. The bottom line is that we are killing our kids, albeit slowly and softly. It is our responsibility to reverse these trends and give our kids a chance at having happy, healthy lives.

I will close with this tongue-in-cheek ironic observation. You want to know how to spot a kid at a playground, mall, or school and determine if he or she is a good kid or bad kid? You cannot tell by their clothes, demeanor or attitude. Just look and see if they are fat or skinny. If he or she is fat, then they are probably good kids. If they are skinny, they are most likely bad kids. And how do I know this? Well, it is simple.

Fat children are eating all their dinners, are behaving, are doing their homework, so they get their reward. A dessert, an ice cream cone, or a candy bar might be awarded.

Meanwhile, the bad kids who lie, cheat, steal or don't finish their plate get no desserts and, thus, no sugar. Poor kids: they are skinny, but ironically, they are the healthy ones and probably have more energy to do their mischievous deeds.

You may be smiling, but think about it. Go to a mall and watch those good kids' smiling faces getting their dopamine rush as they lick their ice cream cones, guzzle their sodas, and munch on their giant cookies. It is a ritual practiced throughout the world.

Sugar is the ultimate parenting tool since society no longer lets us spank our kids. Society now allows us to poison our kids with sugar to make them behave. And the trends are getting worse.

I hope this is not a prophecy, but who knows what the picture will be in another 20 years as the fourth generation of sugar-addicted babies are being born? Will all births be by Cesarean because babies are too big to come through the womb? Will the babies reject their formulas in favor of a Coca Cola? Will we need beds instead of cribs for these massive infants? Will the babies need insulin shots? You may think this is crazy, but talk to a pediatrician and ask him or her what trends he or she is seeing.

To keep from killing our kids the parents must start now setting the example and taking poison out of their diets. Motivation for quitting sugar and fructose must come from all fronts, and hopefully the ultimate turning point will be that we decide to save our children, not kill them.

CHAPTER 15
THE INCREDIBLE LOST OPPORTUNITY TO MAKE PEOPLE HEALTHY: COVID

D o you remember where you were when you first read or heard about Covid? I recall reading something toward the end of 2019 about some new virus breakout in China—something having to do with bats or eating bats from some market in Wuhan. However, I was not particularly alarmed as I recall the many panics and false alarms for numerous viruses that have never affected my life. Viruses like swine flu, SARS, MERS, Ebola, bird flu, this flu, that flu, etc. Now the bat flu. None had ever affected me or the way that I have lived and in 78 years, and I have never had a flu shot.

I distinctly remember speaking with a client in Puerto Rico whom I will call Dr. Dan. He had moved there for tax reasons after selling some ER clinics in Texas. Dr. Dan is somewhat detail-oriented, but he is a smart guy who was crunching some numbers as Covid cases were being reported in China and were spreading in February 2020.

I won't bore you or try to explain what Dr. Dan conveyed to me by phone as my last statistics class was in 1969, so I am a bit hazy on the subject. But I recall him discussing many ratios and numbers such as Pearson's correlation coefficient, the association between observed and predicted values, relative infection ratios, case fatality ratios, and R0s (a mathematical term that indicates how infectious a disease is). If R0 > 1 the disease could become a pandemic. Dr. Dan was saying the R0 was greater than 1 for Covid. As Dr. Dan was talking I felt a pending sense of doom coming over me.

My bottom line takeaway was simply that this virus was spreading faster and quicker than what was being reported by the so-called "health authorities," including the WHO (World Health Organization) and numerous governments, including the United States NIH (National Institute of Health) and China. According to Dr. Dan, Covid was spreading exponentially, and it was going to have a serious negative global impact. It was a true pandemic in the making.

This certainly got my attention and prompted me to do some research as to how this virus might affect me if I caught it. What became immediately obvious was that Covid is an inflammatory virus that has the most serious implications for attacking persons who are already in an inflamed state—in other words, those who are obese, diabetic or pre-diabetic, or have pre-existing coronary disease or metabolic syndrome. So, in my mind the best way to protect oneself from Covid was to have a strong immune system and not to be in an inflamed state.

I knew I was in good shape in that regard. All my blood work was in tolerance, my glucose levels were low, my blood pressure was 120/80, and I was not pre-diabetic. I also knew that part of optimizing my immune system, besides eating healthy food, was to get plenty of exercise and sunshine and 7-8 hours of sleep each night. Vitamin D was especially important, and even in March 2020 there was data being released advising the taking of Vitamin D to protect oneself from Covid.

In the middle of March 2020, Colombia announced a Covid lockdown and seemed to be following the United States' lead and Dr. Anthony Fauci's advice. I was concerned because Colombia was going to close the gyms, which meant no more workouts with weights or cardio since the lockdown extended to not being able to leave your home except to go one day a week for groceries or medicine. Fortunately, I was able to purchase some dumbbells two days before the lockdown so that, every other day, I did some weight work, including push ups and sit ups, in my apartment and on my balcony. Additionally, I started walking on alternate days from my parking garage up a slight incline to the front of my apartment and back for an hour. My porteros (doormen) said nothing and did not report me to the authorities. I upped my intake of Vitamin D, got plenty of sunshine from my balcony, did all my exercises, and made a point to eat even better than ever, with daily salads and limited carbs. In fact, I posted photos on Facebook of my many different salad combinations that I could come up with, which included foods such as avocados, olives, lettuce, cheeses, tomatoes, radishes, cilantro, sun-dried tomatoes, fish, shrimp, chicken, steak, guacamole, onion, carrots, celery, cucumber, lime juice, olive oil, and some occasional fruit. I kept trying different combinations to keep it healthy and interesting.

My life actually stayed pretty normal as my maid was able to come by taxi once a week as well as my manicurist and the gal who cuts my hair. The only things I could not do were go on a vacation, go to live sporting events, or dine at local restaurants.

However, the big event that occurred was the rollout of the *vaccines*. Wow, panic and confusion. Which one should one get? The list of choices was lengthy and included Johnson & Johnson, Moderna, Pfizer, AstraZeneca, Sinopharm, Novavax, and others. Then there were the concerning rumors, many suppressed by the mainstream media. There were reports of some severe side effects, blood clotting, and that some vaccines had not gone through the normal long-term rigorous FDA blind pool testing on humans. And then there was the debate about the efficacy of the new mRNA technology being adopted in the Pfizer and Moderna vaccines. This was especially interesting as it was so new and novel. Was it an incredible breakthrough, or were millions of people going to be human guinea pigs and, in ten to twenty years, see if the experiment had worked or not?

It seemed like there was tremendous pressure being brought to bear on doctors and healthcare authorities to push the vaccines upon the populations in many countries, Colombia included. Thus, getting advice from doctors who were sort of in the dark plus being pressured was not necessarily the best choice. Thankfully, the Internet gives us the ability to research like never before in history and enables some people to make their own informed choices. I have long since learned that money interests often influence or control the decisions of most countries whether it be about starting wars, creating unhealthy products (like processed foods, tobacco, sugar, etc.), healthcare, or other industries.

The average person thinks the vaccines were free, but they were not. The taxpayer was paying an arm and a leg to pay for all of these different vaccines and the distribution and administration of such. It becomes even more evident when looking at the stock prices of the vaccine companies. It was no surprise vaccines were being pushed so hard. Then there are the conflicts of interest between so many key persons in the NIH, CDC, FDA, and other healthcare authorities, who are being compensated or even hired by Big Pharma.

So, with all of this in mind I made my big decision to not get vaccinated. And then the calls started. Over a six-month period in Colombia, I received four calls from EPS (the national health insurance program in Colombia) asking me to get vaccinated. At 77 years of age at that time, I was in the high-risk group, so they were encouraging me to get vaccinated. I was impressed that they were organized enough, and cared enough, to call me. Their heart was in the right place, but I had made my decision and each time I said the same thing: "muchas gracias para tu llamada pero no tengo no interesa en la vacuna." In other words, thanks but no thanks, I am taking a pass on the vaccine.

In essence, I was betting my life on my decision. A lot of folks my age who were in nursing homes and other places were dropping like flies. One older person in my building in Medellin succumbed to Covid. But I was convinced that this flu would not take me down. My health, my diet, my immune system, and my exercise regimen told me that I would be OK if I got the flu. And then, in April 2021, I got Covid.

It was a Friday and I noticed my energy was a bit lower than normal, so I canceled a date that I had for that night. I did go out Saturday night for dinner and seemed OK. Then Sunday, I canceled another date as my energy was down again. On Monday I got tested, and I tested positive for Covid 19. I stayed at home for the week and avoided contact with anyone and waited for the Covid to "do its thing." I took some aspirin a couple of nights as I felt a little feverish, but not much. I had almost no dry cough, no headache, no aches or pains, and no sneezing. I did experience a little brain fog, my energy was down, and I slept a bit more than usual. I may have lost my sense of taste one night, but I am not sure. Overall, it was, for me, less intrusive than a common cold. I have had no after-effects that I am aware of from the dreaded long Covid. Everything was quickly back to normal, and I felt vindicated in my decision.

In time I became particularly irritated with the pressure being put on people to get vaccinated. Washington DC did their standard trick of keeping us divided and distracted, creating two camps of the vaxxers and anti-vaxxers, both waging war on each other. Of course, the money interests, news media and the paid-off government took the side of the vaxxers. Soon the anti-vaxxers started losing their jobs, could not eat at restaurants, could not fly or travel internationally, could not play in certain sports events, etc. They were treated like lepers and incurred the righteousness of the vaccinated. It became more and more ridiculous how the anti-vaxxers were being discriminated against.

Soon, however, the uncovering of the vaccine lies/bad information began. It started with the myth that getting vaccinated would prevent you from getting Covid. This got blown up when vaccinated people got Covid a second and third time. Even President Biden got it twice. The next lie was that if you are vaccinated you would not spread Covid. The vaxxers were accusing anti-vaxxers of being horrible people for spreading Covid and possibly killing people. It seemed the anti-vaxxers were just shy of being satanic as they were accused of spreading Covid to the elderly and killing grandma and grandpa. Then this diatribe became further complicated as it became evident that vaccinated people were spreading Covid as well. Another tale had to do with wearing almost worthless cloth and paper masks. Unless you were wearing a hazmat suit or a special N95 mask, the masks were virtually ineffective in protecting you from getting or spreading Covid. The masks did, however, affect your respiration and did trap bacteria.

To date, the human toll of the pandemic lockdown is almost immeasurable in terms of setting back the education of children, the rise of drug use and alcohol, the increase in depression and suicide, the break up of marriages, the negative impact on economies and income around the world, and many other issues. But, to me, the saddest thing was the lost opportunity to help the world, especially in the United States, the most obese country in the world with its 128 million diabetics and pre-diabetics. The United States suffered the most Covid deaths in absolute terms and as a percentage of the population. Anybody can go to the Internet and research the most obese countries in the world and the percent of deaths due to Covid. Then do a simple correlation and regression analysis and see the link between Covid deaths and overweight people. The latest numbers indicate that the United States, with 4.2% of the world's population, had 16% of Covid deaths.

What is wrong with this picture? What should have been done?

COVID: THE WORLD WAS WAITING FOR ADVICE

Well, Covid was a great motivator, and it had a captive audience waiting for advice.

The health authorities of the world were able to scare the world into becoming like a herd of sheep. Wear ineffective masks, stay indoors, close the gyms, get no sunshine, avoid human contact, shut down schools, close businesses, etc. The result was that Fauci and the US government's advice made us sicker. No vitamin D from sunshine, no exercise, no walks on the beach, no being able to go outdoors…and the worst part was that processed-food sales went up by 25%, which made the general populace even sicker, more inflamed, and more vulnerable to having a negative Covid outcome.

THE LOST OPPORTUNITY WAS THIS!

Dr. Fauci, the NIH, CDC, and the WHO should have said that the best way to prevent a negative Covid outcome is this: quit eating sugar, processed food, soft drinks, candy, ice cream, desserts, white bread, vegetable cooking oils, and high-glycemic veggies like potatoes and white rice. Start exercising. Get seven to eight hours of sleep. Eat more fruits, vegetables, eggs, fish, and healthy meats. Take Vitamin D and other similar supplements and vitamins. Covid could have been a great motivator for people to lose weight,exercise, eat real food, and get healthy to reduce their bodies' inflammation and chronic disease. Of course, this message would have been predicated with a warning that if you cannot, or will not, take these life-saving tips, then you should consider getting vaccinated so as to help lessen the life-threatening effects of Covid. Each person should have been allowed to consult his or her informed physician as to whether the vaccine is a good idea or not and then weigh the possible negative effects and/or risks of the vaccine vs. the risk of what Covid might do to one's health and longevity when they caught it.

But of course, this was not done. The opportunity to tell America and the rest of the world that sugar is bad for your health was lost. How much of this was due to the greed and self-serving money interests of Big Pharma, paid-off politicians, and other money interests will be debated over time. But what a shame that the opportunity was missed. The herds were lined up ready and waiting for their supposed good medical advice. What they got instead was a travesty as opposed to what they should have received: the truth about sugar. The results were that sugar, combined with Covid, was not killing anybody softly; it was a tragic outcome. Instead of creating a healthier society, we ended up with a sicker society.

THEY SHOULD HAVE NAMED IT THE SUGAR FLU

The facts are that the pre-existing conditions of diabetes, obesity, cardiovascular problems, and high blood pressure are found in the majority of Covid 19 deaths. All of these conditions are markers for sugar, processed food and high-fructose corn syrup (HFCS) consumption. The top two countries with the highest death rates are also the top two consumers per capita of sugar and HFCS (United States and Brazil). Conversely, countries with the lowest BMI (body mass index - a measure of obesity) had the lowest percentage of death rates. This includes many SE Asia countries, like Japan and Vietnam, which rank near the bottom of the world's BMI rankings. Their diets have very little sugar, HFCS or processed foods. They should rename Covid 19 the "Sugar Flu" as it was killing the sugar, processed-food and HFCS consumers. But the news media and politicians will not connect those dots because of entrenched financial interests and their lobbyists. The bottom line is that, if you are healthy, Covid most likely will be more like a typical flu with normal outcomes. However, if you are a heavy sugar consumer and eat a lot of processed foods, then you may need to take precautions. So, the real story here is the poor diets of the US, Mexico, UK, Brazil, Great Britain, etc. Covid 19 was perhaps nature's wake-up call to eat real food and quit sugar. What a shame that nobody was telling us this.

CHAPTER 16
THE TOBACCO TEMPLATE FOR SUGAR REDUCTION

My editor suggested that I leave out this paragraph because it is not about sugar. The reason that I am overruling her is because of feedback from ordinary people like yourself. Over the past seven years, I have found it is difficult to get people to even believe that sugar is destroying their health, but when I finally get a convert, they say, "What's the use? It can never happen. There is no way to change the system."

Well my answer is, yes there is, and the Tobacco Template is the answer.

I am probably older than 95% of the readers of this book. As such you have missed some interesting things from the early days of my life, such as rotary telephones, drive-in movie theaters, Pez candy, soda shops, conical bras, and black-and-white TVs.

When I was a very young kid in the early 1950s, I vividly remember watching TV in black and white when a television commercial interrupted the Western that I was watching. The commercial went as follows: a doctor walks on stage in his white smock with a stethoscope around his neck while smoking, and obviously enjoying, a cigarette. A voice-over says, "More doctors prefer Camels," and then the doctor would extol the virtues of smoking, claiming it gives you more energy, pleasure, and relaxation.

Related campaigns emphasized that "Luckies" would help consumers—especially women, their new market—stay slim, since they could "Reach for a Lucky instead of a sweet."

Touting surveys conducted by "three leading independent research organizations," one typical advertisement proclaimed that according to "nationwide" surveys of 113,597 doctors "from every branch of medicine," Camel was the brand smoked by most respondents.

There were catchy slogans such as, "Winston tastes good like a cigarette should." Also, "LSMFT (Luckies Mean Finer Tobacco)," "I'd walk a mile for a Camel," and "Come to Marlboro country."

There was also a commercial with this claim: "20,679 Physicians say 'Luckies are less irritating'," which featured a white-haired, white-coated doctor with a reassuring smile.

We were inundated with pleasurable ads from Phillip Morris, Marlboro, Chesterfield, Old Gold, Pall Mall, Salem, and numerous other brands. Many of these brands were being touted by our biggest influencers, including movie stars, athletes like Mickey Mantle, news broadcasters, doctors, researchers and even Santa Claus, all enjoying a smoke.

I remember later buying fake candy cigarettes that had leading brand names. It was little wonder that I later became a smoker, joining almost half of the United States in doing so. Over time, information and research clearly showed that smoking was bad for you and could lead to lung cancer and heart disease. On Jan 1, 1971 the last TV commercial for cigarettes ran on *The Johnny Carson Show*.

Over the next 20 years the anti-smoking bandwagon gained momentum, with cigarettes being restricted to minors and taken out of schools. There were public service and government warnings; newspapers, magazines, and TV ran anti-smoking ads and coverage; and doctors stopped touting cigarettes and, in most cases, quit themselves. Very importantly, warning labels were required to be printed clearly on all cigarette packages. Later, restaurants, sports venues, public spaces, airplanes, etc. banned smoking and soon, it became uncool. It literally took about 30-40 years to get US smoking down from 42% to under 14%.

As I think about it now, it is incredible that it took this long to provide informed consent to the United States populace and the world, and to tell the truth about the obvious perils of smoking.

This clearly illustrates what can happen when a harmful addictive substance like nicotine can be used to make billions of dollars in profits for unscrupulous corporations who only care about profits, not your well-being. For many years, Big Tobacco had a free run on advertising, duping the medical community, and avoiding negative press. Lobbyists paid off the politicians, so there was no governmental scrutiny, no public education, no warnings, etc. It took a long time to finally put tobacco in its place in the United States and most developed countries with the intended results of lowering smoking by 400% or more.

I believe there is a parallel between harmful, addictive tobacco and harmful, addictive sugar. Tobacco has given us a template for drastically reducing smoking, albeit taking a long time. However, Big Sugar is a much more formidable foe with deeper pockets and a much less obvious poison to peddle.

Speaking of peddlers, did you ever wonder what Big Tobacco did when they saw the handwriting on the wall in the 1980s?

Big Tobacco did not sit on its hands. The first thing they did was to start more aggressively marketing to second- and third-world countries—those lesser-developed countries, where cash-starved governments were willing to look the other way. Cigarette consumption has spiked dramatically in many of these countries. Big Tobacco expanded product lines including vaping, e-cigarettes, smokeless tobacco, and snuff. In the US they even raised prices on the hopelessly addicted to maintain their margins. Perhaps their biggest move was to start investing and to take over food companies whose featured product lines contain, you guessed it, *sugar*.

Can sugar be as addictive as cigarettes? The answer is yes. According to a study by the University of Florida, sugary foods can be as addictive as nicotine and cocaine. Their study found that people with obesity were drawn to images of junk food, in the same way cocaine addicts were drawn to images of white powder.[1]

In the 1980s, Big Tobacco was prominent in the takeover of Kraft Foods, General Foods, and Nabisco, which ended up being the biggest leveraged buy-out (LBO) in that decade. Once again Big Tobacco could start its aggressive marketing campaigns, especially those geared toward our kids.

Unlike cigarettes, sugary foods are often widely available in schools, hospitals, and prisons. As of 2022, the law is still on the side of food manufacturers. Most US states, for example, have yet to pass a single law taxing soft drinks.

A former tobacco control researcher stated, "I will proudly raise my right hand and declare: Big Food/Big Tobacco executives are like The Terminator. They will not stop."[2]

Though both food and tobacco companies have been notorious marketers to children, they both like to lecture parents. In the 1990s, RJ Reynolds Tobacco Company noted, "It is the responsibility of every parent to encourage their children to make proper choices about lifestyle decisions." It's not the role of the federal government to discourage kids from smoking, they went on to say. In 2011, McDonald's CEO Jim Skinner said, "It is up to [kids] to choose and their parents to choose, and it is their responsibility to do so."

Joe Camel, the cartoon animal used to attract children to cigarettes, was retired in 1997, under pressure from state attorneys general (AGs). A master settlement agreement between the AGs and the tobacco industry eliminated much of that industry's advertising to children, and even disbanded the Tobacco Institute, an aggressive industry-lobbying force. But the food industry still uses cartoon characters to market disease-causing products to children, and food industry trade groups still devote millions to block progress and defend the status quo.

Big Tobacco and Big Food are now separate divisions, but the playbook is much the same. How the game ends up is up to us. In essence, Big Tobacco has joined Big Sugar with its aggressive marketing techniques, misinformation campaigns, and heavy lobby spending to keep governments under control.[3]

Thanks to the Internet, the public has a much better chance of creating a grassroots movement to get the truth about sugar into the public mainstream so people can make informed choices. It can be done as we have the tobacco template as a model for achieving success in reducing consumption of a harmful addictive substance, nicotine.

The anti-sugar movement is alive and well, and, as Dr. Lustig has stated, we are in year ten of a 30-year fight to reach the position of informed consent about sugar. Along with that I would hope to see truth in labeling for sugar; have it taken out of schools; limit access to minors; impose aggressive taxation; launch public service announcements; have the news media jump aboard; place restrictions on Big Sugar lobbyists; provide mandatory nutritional training for all doctors, dentists and medical professionals; offer insurance coverage for preventative medicine, and use many other related measures to combat sugar consumption.

CHAPTER 17
THE HEALTHY BIG THREE: REAL FOOD, EXERCISE, AND SLEEP

This chapter is short and, in some ways, the most important chapter. It is a simple solution to what ails us. It is what our grandmothers told us and what our doctors sometimes give lip service to. It is so simple, so why don't we embrace the Healthy Big Three?

Part of the problem is a simple credo that has emerged in the American psyche, which is that there is a pill for everything. We all want a magic pill to make us healthy and happy, to lose weight, cure our disease, help us sleep, and provide the benefits of exercise without exercising. Do you think for one minute that Big Pharma might have something to do with this so-called panacea? Big Pharma is the entity most responsible for legions of doctors to be trained to prescribe pills to treat our symptoms instead of treating the cause. And as discussed previously, 75% of the time, the cause can be linked to not eating real food, and eating sugar and sugar-added foods like processed foods.

Hopefully, by now you have some appreciation about how important eating real food is. Dr. Lustig's mantra is: every time you put something into your mouth, ask yourself, "am I protecting my liver and feeding my gut?" Dr. Lustig notes that there is no pill that takes the place of the positive metabolic effects of eating real food. We may not like the concept that food is medicine, but it is. It is a better medicine than any pill we could take.

Eating real food supports all eight of our metabolic cellular functions, and exercise supports five of them. What a health team this is when we do it, but how sad it is when we do not. Importantly, eating crap and not exercising have a dastardly impact on sleep, the third member of the Big Three. Sleep is just as important to good health as is eating real food and exercising. Optimally, seven to eight hours of natural sleep delivers the best health outcomes.

Examples of negative health outcomes of too little sleep are as follows:

- On October 18, 2022, *CNN Health* reported a large new study that provides evidence that people 50 and older who sleep five hours or less at night have a greater risk of developing multiple chronic diseases as they age.
- They faced a 30% higher risk that they would develop multiple chronic diseases over time than those who slept at least seven hours a night. At age 60, it was a 32% increased risk, and at 70, it was a 40% greater risk.
- Diseases with a higher risk included diabetes, cancer, coronary heart disease, stroke, heart failure, chronic obstructive pulmonary disease, chronic kidney disease, liver disease, depression, dementia, mental disorders, Parkinson's, and arthritis.
- Sleep is a restorative process that, among other things, produces and regulates hormones in the body.
- Hormones regulate things like appetite, metabolism, sex drive, blood pressure and heart rate, body temperature, and circadian rhythms.
- A recent Ted Talk indicated that upon losing one hour of sleep, the risk of a heart attack goes up by 24% the next day, and that is reversed when one gains one hour of sleep. Also, at only four hours sleep there is a 70% drop of natural killer cell activity (the cells that support our immune system). There is a direct link to cancer and sleep deprivation. In essence, short sleep equals a short life.

Sugar and processed foods can interrupt sleep as follows:

- Foods high in sugar and processed carbohydrates cause a rapid increase in blood sugar levels. This triggers a corresponding release of insulin, which helps regulate blood sugar. However, this process can lead to a sudden drop in blood sugar later on, resulting in a state of hypoglycemia. These fluctuations in blood sugar can disrupt your sleep, causing you to wake up during the night or experience difficulty falling asleep.
- Processed foods are low in fiber and high in unhealthy fats, which can lead to digestive problems such as indigestion, acid reflux, and discomfort. These issues can make it challenging to get comfortable and fall asleep peacefully.
- Many processed foods, especially those with added sugars or artificial additives, contain stimulants like caffeine and certain food additives. These substances can interfere with your ability to fall asleep or stay asleep, leading to disrupted sleep patterns.
- Relying heavily on processed foods can result in a lack of essential nutrients like vitamins, minerals, and antioxidants. Nutritional deficiencies can affect sleep quality and overall health, as various nutrients play a role in regulating sleep-wake cycles and promoting relaxation.
- Consistently consuming sugary and processed foods can contribute to weight gain and obesity. Excessive weight gain, particularly around the neck area, can increase the risk of developing sleep apnea, a sleep disorder characterized by interrupted breathing during sleep. Sleep apnea disrupts sleep patterns and can lead to poor sleep quality.

To promote better sleep, it is generally recommended to adopt a balanced and nutritious diet that includes whole foods, plenty of fruits and vegetables, lean proteins, and complex carbohydrates. Additionally, reducing or eliminating your intake of sugary and processed foods, especially close to bedtime, can positively impact your sleep.

Who is the primary beneficiary for sleeping disorders? The companies who sell sleeping pills, Big Pharma. In the year 2021 profits from sleeping pills and aids in the US were $64.1 billion. This amount is nothing to snooze about but could be drastically reduced if people ate real food and exercised. Granted, there are a number of other factors that can affect sleep such as erratic schedules, noise, alcohol, environmental factors, taking stimulants before bedtime, and stress, but the impact of these can be lessened if you are eating right and exercising.

Stress is the wild card and is the unwanted, uninvited guest of the Big Three. Stress can affect sleep, disrupt exercise, and cause binge eating of bad foods and excess drinking. All of this is bad enough, but stress also brings its ugly uncle, cortisol, to the party.

Cortisol, often referred to as the "stress hormone," is produced by the adrenal glands in response to stress or perceived threats.

High levels of cortisol can suppress the immune system, making you more susceptible to infections, illnesses, and inflammatory conditions. It can also hinder the body's ability to heal wounds and recover from injuries.

Chronic elevation of cortisol levels has been linked to an increased risk of cardiovascular issues. It can contribute to high blood pressure, atherosclerosis (hardening of the arteries), and an increased risk of heart disease and stroke.

Cortisol can influence appetite, cravings, and fat storage. Prolonged elevation of cortisol levels can lead to increased appetite, particularly for high-calorie foods, and result in weight gain, especially in the abdominal area. Cortisol can also affect the body's metabolism, potentially leading to metabolic disturbances and insulin resistance.

Excess cortisol can interfere with memory, concentration, and overall cognitive function. It may contribute to difficulties with learning, attention, and decision-making. Chronic stress and elevated cortisol levels have also been associated with an increased risk of developing conditions like anxiety and depression.

Cortisol follows a diurnal pattern, with higher levels in the morning to help wake you up and lower levels in the evening to promote sleep. However, chronic stress can disrupt this natural rhythm, leading to elevated cortisol levels at night. This can make it difficult to fall asleep or stay asleep, resulting in sleep disturbances and insomnia.

Elevated cortisol levels can affect digestion and nutrient absorption, potentially leading to digestive issues such as stomach ulcers, acid reflux, irritable bowel syndrome (IBS), and appetite changes.

It's important to note that cortisol is a natural and necessary hormone in the body, and short-term increases in cortisol during acute stress situations are normal. However, chronic stress and sustained high cortisol levels will have detrimental effects on overall health, as noted above.

The bottom line is when you combine stress with chronic disease, negative outcomes can and will be accelerated. The best way to combat stress is by eating real food, exercising, and sleeping right.

I have been very fortunate to have come up with the idea that when I am stressed from work, an emotional entanglement, have fear about something, money problems, etc., I actually increase my exercise regimen. It is amazing how that helps to lower stress. Additionally, the increased exercise helps me sleep better, again lowering the stress and allowing me to live to fight another day. I have counseled many friends over the years that when things are going bad, this is a great opportunity to create something positive, like exercising more, getting into great shape, and looking better physically.

The sad thing for many people is when stress is high there is a temptation to indulge in comfort foods and actually increase our intake of sugary products, ice cream, soft drinks, pies, desserts, pizza, chips, candy, booze, and drugs. This plays into the hand of stress, exacerbating the situation even more and can result in making our chronic diseases even worse. It can be a vicious cycle that is best thwarted by ramping up the Big Three: eating real food even more strictly, increasing our exercise regimen, and getting seven to eight hours of sleep.

Do not let stress be the catalyst that kills you.

Of course, as previously noted, incorporating The Big Healthy Three into your life not only helps you prevent metabolic disease, but it also helps combat and mitigate stress.

CHAPTER 18
KISS (KEEP IT SIMPLE STUPID)

What is KISS and why is it being included in a book detailing the perils of sugar consumption?

KISS, an acronym for "Keep it simple, stupid!", is a design principle noted by the US Navy in 1960. KISS states that designs and / or systems should be as simple as possible. Wherever possible, complexity should be avoided in a system—as simplicity guarantees the greatest levels of user acceptance and interaction.

So how does this relate to avoiding sugar?

As noted earlier in this book, the Sugar Industry likes to keep us confused and distracted with all of its misinformation, mistruths, and misguided influence. The general public is not only bombarded with mistruths, but the real truth is also hidden from us. The US government is not issuing warnings or public service announcements, the news media is basically silent, the doctors are not on top of it as they are basically being trained to prescribe pills to treat the symptoms of sugar addiction, and the US sick-care system has no motivation for preventive medicine. And the list goes on.

DIETS KEEP US DISTRACTED

Then there are diets. Yes, so many diets are being proposed that it almost boggles the mind. I have no evidence to show that the Sugar Industry is behind the diet industry, but they must love it more than a hot fudge sundae. Take, for example, the many diet choices that the public has such as the following:

- The vegan diet
- Low-carb diets
- The Dukan diet
- The ultra-low-fat diet
- The Atkins diet
- The HCG diet
- The zone diet
- The paleo diet
- The blood type diet
- The South Beach diet
- The Mediterranean diet
- Raw food diet
- Oprah Winfrey diets
- Vegetarian diet
- DASH diet
- Weight Watchers
- Noom diet
- Pescatarian diet
- Ornish diet
- MIND diet
- Nordic diet
- Keto diet
- Beverly Hills diet
- Nutrisystem diet
- Pritikin diet
- Scarsdale medical diet
- Jenny Craig
- Macrobiotic diet

- Juice fasting
- Intermittent fasting [1]

Many people try multiple diets because they have no success with their initial diet programs. So, diets offer many choices and hopes, and can be confusing. And with new ones coming up every year, they clearly violate KISS.

DO DIETS WORK?

If diets truly worked, the 72-billion-dollar diet industry would tank overnight because there would be no repeat customers.

According to the latest weight-loss research, 95% of dieters end up regaining the weight they lost within two years. Calorie-restricting diets are often successful at helping people lose weight, but they're very unsuccessful at helping people maintain that weight loss. [2]

Each year, more than 50% of American adults try to lose weight. The diet industry in the United States makes more than $70 billion per year. (Yes, that says "billion.") Yet research shows that diets don't work: 90 to 97% of people who lose weight through dieting will regain it back within two to five years. When you restrict or limit certain types of food, or cut back on the amount of food you eat, your body gets the message that you are starving, so it switches into survival mode. It doesn't matter if you are surrounded by enough food to feed you for weeks. Your body is still biologically wired as it was centuries ago when food was truly scarce, and the ability to store extra calories as fat and burn fewer calories at rest was a genetic survival mechanism. [3]

That means that now, any threat of restriction or food scarcity (like a new diet or setting food rules) feels to your body like starvation is coming. And when your body senses starvation, it does everything it can to try to keep you alive and to keep you within your set-point weight range.

Your body does this in a variety of ways, including the following:

- Decreasing your metabolic rate (aka, the number of calories your body needs each day to stay alive)

- Decreasing thyroid activity (which is involved in regulating metabolism)
- Decreasing levels of your fullness hormones
- Increasing levels of your hunger hormones
- Increasing your cravings for calorie-dense foods[4]

There are plenty more scientific and medical references as to why diets do not work, so this is not really debatable. The challenge is certainly significant, and this is where KISS comes in.

With KISS we only have to concentrate on one thing: quit eating sugar and the stuff we put into our bodies that converts into sugar. With this program we are not restricting calories. We can eat all we want until we are full. Our body chemistry will respond well to this since with limited or no sugar, and in turn lower glucose and minimal insulin being released, leptin will do its job, we will feel satiated, and less dopamine will be released thus eliminating eating binges. As a result of minimal glucose in our systems, we now have the ability to burn fat as the body needs to do this to add glucose to the bloodstream. Our metabolic rate will increase during this process. Our "fat switch" will not be triggered. The best news of all is that, by eliminating the addictive poison, sugar, we will crave it less and less to the point we do not miss it at all. I know from personal experience that I do not miss, want, or even think about desserts or sweets any more.

The key with KISS is to jumpstart the program as will be noted in the next chapter. However, KISS will have its challenges as follows:

- There are more than 56 different names for sugar, so we need to be aware of them and eliminate them from our eating regimens.
- These different names for sugar are on labels in the grocery store, but Big Food makes it difficult to read the labels.
- Perhaps take a magnifying glass with you when shopping; some even have LED lights for better viewing.
- On the other hand, a good rule of thumb is that, if there is a label, there is a good chance it has sugar in it or is a processed food. It is best to be a skeptic when seeing a label.

- 75% of the items in your grocery store have labels and have sugar, convert to sugar, and/or are processed.
- According to a recent CBS News survey, 56% of Americans dine at a restaurant, get take-out, or have a meal delivered two to three times a week.
- Avoid fast food restaurants at all costs, but of course, they are conveniently located on every street corner.
- The idea of healthy restaurants offering sugar-free dining is a new concept that is in its infancy, so one needs to be aware of what is being served. Some healthy options can be found in vegetarian, vegan, keto restaurants and other restaurants offering quality fare.
- Until the US food industry shifts towards healthy eating due to increased demand, it will be incumbent on each of us to find ways of keeping our food interesting and tasty.

So, one of the keys is to keep it interesting so KISS can do its job.

You might have noticed on the list of diets above that intermittent fasting was noted last. Interestingly, this type of fast or diet works well with those giving up sugar because you feel satiated and it is very easy to hold off on your first meal until 1-4 PM. As noted previously, there is research that illustrates that intermittent fasting is good for your immune system and for leading a healthy lifestyle. Sugar eaters will find intermittent fasting almost impossible while sugar haters will have no problem.

To the delight of the Sugar Industry, the messages are mixed, confusing, and often realistic. Plus, the lead in this is not the medical community. The best advice we get from them is to exercise, diet, and eat more fruits and vegetables.

So, when it comes to dieting, how many of us wish to diet and how many of us can do it for a month, six months, a year, a lifetime? Almost nobody but the most fanatical amongst us.

Who among us today wants to be a vegetarian or a vegan or a disciple of an extreme alkaline diet? As much as I admire and appreciate those regimens, I do know how tough it is to adopt them unless our bodies and minds are pre-conditioned for doing such.

Who wants to join Weight Watchers or Jenny Craig, go to meetings, and eat their food? I am not saying they do not work or are not a good cause because they do reduce sugar and carbs in many of their programs. But are they sustainable, and will the general public stay with them?

Then there are the calorie counters. Yikes. Unless you are some type of accountant who loves tracking numbers, counting calories is about as much fun as counting sheep when trying to sleep. Plus, as discussed previously, it is not about the calories, it is about jumpstarting the metabolic process. As I mentioned, I lost 22 pounds in 21 days during my first detox and never counted one calorie and was never hungry for a minute.

And of course, there is exercise. We should all exercise with both cardio and weights for many reasons. But will we have the motivation and energy to do so? We might if we suddenly dropped 10-50 pounds as our energy would go up and the task of exercise would be less daunting. It is all about motivation and momentum. But if you are an overweight couch potato eating carbs and sugar, you are probably the least interested person in the world in going to the gym, drawing stares and giggles as all the muscle-toned attendees stare at your prohibitive pot belly, big butt, and cellulite. However, when we see personal progress and feel better, we tend to jump on board that progress train, and joining a gym, or hiring a personal trainer to jump start us becomes more of a reality.

KISS works. No sugar, exercise (easier when you do not eat sugar), and seven to eight hours of sleep each night (easier when you do not eat sugar), all mean living longer, healthier and happier, and spending less time at the doctor's office.

HOW DO WE IMPLEMENT KISS?

It is simple. For now, just ignore everything above.

I want you to instead write down these five things to *never* eat—ever. If you exclude them from your eating program you will see miracles within your health, energy, and well-being. You will want to start exercising. You will feel like exercising. You might even wish to be a vegetarian. But you will feel like making new healthy choices.

So here goes. Just do not eat these five things and your life will improve dramatically, your health will improve, you will lose weight, your skin will improve to the point you will look 10-15 years younger, and you might even find your libido improving.

DO NOT EAT:

1. Strychnine
2. Rat poison
3. Dead cockroaches
4. Cow feces
5. Sugar

Simple. We can all do it. You can do it. But if you should eat one of these items on this list, which would not injure your health?

If you have been paying attention, it is the dead cockroaches. They are protein and can be metabolized, and they protect the liver and feed the gut. You may wish to microwave or bake them first to kill off any unnecessary bacteria. Perhaps add some seasoning. Just do not eat the sugar.

Once you quit sugar, you will find some interesting other side benefits.

As you withdraw from sugar you will start to lose your craving for sweets, soft drinks, candy, ice cream, etc. Fruits and vegetables will start tasting sweeter to the point you will start craving them and wanting to snack on them instead of forcing yourself to. This is especially important for your children. Interestingly, my desire to eat red meat has decreased. Not that I am against steak, but I prefer to go more for white meats and fish. I do not know why, but I have noticed it, and there is nothing wrong with that.

Your shopping cart will change not only in composition but in cost. Remember that 75% of the items in your supermarket (unless you shop at Whole Foods, health food stores, or organic markets) will be processed foods that will have some form of sugar/fructose in them.

So, your cart will look much different with eggs, meat, chicken, fish, veggies, fruits, nuts, dietary bread, granola, stevia, water with and without carbonation, etc. And your lower tab at the checkout counter will be appreciated as well.

So, go for KISS starting today. Afterwards you can decide if you wish to take it to the next level, but at the very least you have taken a huge step forward that will extend your life, reduce your health care costs, improve your attitude and self-confidence, and, very importantly, stop your family and children from being a part of the fourth generation of sugar addicts in the United States/Canada (or third generation in Europe, Australia and Central/South America, or second generation in Asia and the Middle East).

The choice is yours. It is simple. You now have the tool. Why let the trillion-dollar Sugar Industry destroy your life. Let's turn them into a billion-dollar industry and let them look for other work.

CHAPTER 19
THE ROLE OF SUGAR IN ANTI-AGING AND PREVENTIVE MEDICINE

W hen we are younger, we have a lot of things going for us, but we often lack that special trait called wisdom. This comes with age and experience. Many of us in our younger years believe we are invincible and we live in the moment, not worrying about the future, living longer, or even dying.

A large number of people, as they age into their 50s, 60s, and 70s, start to think about death, wills, and how to live longer. But for many, it is too late as chronic disease has set in, a lot of time is being spent with doctors, taking a variety of pills, and visits to the hospital. For some, it means being confined in an assisted living facility or nursing home. At this point preventative medicine and anti-aging programs are too late.

But for the younger generation and even those who are oldsters, preventative medicine and anti-aging protocols are worth exploring.

PREVENTIVE MEDICINE

A preventive medicine specialist focuses on the health of individuals and defined populations in order to protect, promote, and maintain health and well-being, and to prevent disease, disability, and prema-ture death. As mentioned earlier, less than 2% of the 4.3 trillion USD annual healthcare expenditures in the US are for preventive medicine. The Sugar Industry likes it this way as it fits well into their plans for maximizing revenues and profits.

Princeton Longevity Center NYC, Mayo Clinic, Fountain Life, GoForward.com, and Ways2Well are some examples of clinical practices prescribing and promoting preventive medicine. A recent update on this subject is found in an article titled, "The Longevity Clinic Will See You Now—for $100,000," which notes that these clinics cater to a growing number of people obsessed with fighting aging.[1]

There will be many more of these types of clinics in the future with preventative medicine as a central component, but hopefully getting people off of sugar and processed foods will not be ignored as this is not a big money maker in the preventative medicine field. In fact, getting people off of sugar and processed foods should always be the simplest, quickest, and least costly first step in preventative medicine.

ANTI-AGING

David Andrew Sinclair, AO is an Australian-American biologist and academic known for his research on aging and epigenetics. Sinclair is a professor of genetics at Harvard Medical School and is the co-director of its Paul F. Glenn Center for Biology of Aging Research. At age 54, David Sinclair has the appearance of a young man in his late 20s or early 30s.

I first heard of David Sinclair during a Joe Rogan broadcast. I was fascinated by his comments on how to reverse aging and some of the supplements that he took, such as nicotinamide mononucleotide (NMN), resveratrol, and Metformin. After studying this more and reading Sinclair's book *Lifespan*, I added his supplements to my vitamin program (although I have since quit taking Metformin). The basic ideas of anti-aging are to start early and nip this aging thing in the bud. For me, starting at age 73+ to quit sugar and processed foods, and after years of pretty heavy drinking, it was a bit late to think about the possibilities of this new field of anti-aging, which promotes the idea of living well after 100 years of age, healthily, happily and actively. I know of a number of younger people today who are on strict anti-aging protocols who plan to live to be 120-130 years of age. The science and technology are there, and I do not doubt it will happen. But it is a bit late for me, and my goal is simply to make it to 100 years of age, healthily, happily, and actively.

A major player who has cast his two cents' worth is Tony Robbins, and his recent book, *Life Force*, co-authored by Peter Diamandis, MD and Robert Hariri, MD, Ph.D. What I liked about this book is it is a great up-to-date summary of all the many anti-aging protocols, science, and developments that are occurring today. *Life Force* explores hormone replacement therapy, peptides, stem cell treatments, supplements, sleep, gene splicing, bio technology, the gut microbiome, etc.

As I read *Life Force*, I kept waiting to get to the section of the most important part of anti-aging, the very thing that ages us prematurely and has a browning effect on our cells, that ages our skin, that causes us to die prematurely—and that, of course, is sugar.

My biggest complaint regarding *Life Force* is that this critical and most important first step to anti-aging (quitting sugar and processed foods) is buried on page 492, with a quote from Dr. Robert Lustig, as follows:

> *The Seductive Dangers of Our Food Environment - sugar is now the most ubiquitous foodstuff worldwide, and has been added to virtually every processed food, limiting consumer choice and the ability to avoid it. Approximately 80% of the 6 million consumer packaged foods in the U.S. have added caloric sweeteners.*
>
> *-ROBERT LUSTIG, MD*

That was about all there was. Not a chapter, nor a full page, just a quick paragraph on this critical subject, about the life-ruining effects of consuming sugar.

I do not mean to be critical of Tony Robbins and *Life Force*, as this is an excellent book, but there was the hook at the end, and that is the promotion of Fountain Life, the new preventative medicine program being launched in several US locations, in which Tony has partnered with some doctors and healthcare specialists. To me, it is a bit expensive for the average person and there may be more cost-effective competitors, but any preventative medicine is better than none, no matter what the cost, so in that regard I wish Fountain Life success. But I have to wonder if *Life Force* could have done its readers a service by saying that the first step for any preventative medicine program is to *quit sugar*.

Of course, nobody makes any money saying that. Hopefully, that is not the reason for omitting that advice in *Life Force*.

Along these lines, I will tell you a funny story about stem cells. I live two blocks from probably the biggest stem cell clinic in Colombia, BioExcellerator. It has become sort of famous as several MMA fighters and some athletes have been singing its praises. Just after they opened about four years ago, I visited them to see if it might fit into my newfound health and desire to live longer and better. For about $10,000 USD, I could have been injected with about 100 million placenta-based stem cells. They even had an anaerobic chamber where you can watch Netflix as a part of the procedures. I decided to take a pass as I had nothing wrong with me, no sports injuries, and my health seemed great.

Fast-forward several years, the cost for the basic BioExcellerator program is up to $30,000 USD, and three different friends of mine had come to Medellin for stem cell treatments for such things as shoulder and knee pain, hair replacement, EDS, and some other items. After their treatments, their overall results over time seemed to be neutral, no strong recommendations from any of them, and no real endorsements. But nothing really negative. They seemed to be comfortable with giving the true results more time to appear. However, the one important thing I will remember is from my friend—I will call him Bob —who told me this amazing story.

Bob said one month before coming to Medellin for the BioExcellerator treatment, he was contacted by a gorgeous dietician who told Bob to start a program for 30 days in order to maximize the results of the stem cell treatments. When Bob arrived in Medellin, he told me how good he felt and, in fact, it was the best he had felt in years. This was before the stem cell treatments even started.

Well, you could have knocked me over with a feather when I reviewed Bob's suggested pre-treatment program. The dietician had taken Bob off of sugar, booze, and processed foods, and he was experiencing a major health transformation. I have since wondered if some of BioExcellerator's patients might be confusing the success from detoxing with their stem cell treatments?

This is the perfect segue into our final chapter—your very important next step to great health and experiencing your own life-saving personal miracle.

CHAPTER 20
THE PATH TO YOUR PERSONAL MIRACLE AND NEW GREAT HEALTH IS SIMPLE AND FREE

DR. RASA NIKANJAM'S 21-DAY DETOX PROGRAM

I f you have read this far, congratulations! Perhaps you are not a hopelessly addicted sugar addict, and you have an open mind about improving your own health or that of your family or people you care about. On the other hand, maybe you just skipped the previous 19 chapters and jumped to the end to save time. In either case, it does not matter.

What does matter is that you want to improve your health and live longer, healthier, and happier. If this is your intention, then here is your no-cost solution.

You need to do the same 21-day detox that I did. It is just 21 days of your life—you can do this. But I want to add a very important caveat.

Do not do the detox if you are not seriously committed, or if you will be tempted to cheat for any reason at all. If you cheat, you will not experience the miracle, and you will never believe in the truth that sugar and processed foods are killing you softly.

I say this in all sincerity. My life was saved by this miracle and I want to give back. I want everybody to experience what I experienced, and if I can save just one life, then writing this book will have been worth it. With this in mind, here is the program that saved my life and can save yours as well:

DR. RASA NIKANJAM'S 21-DAY DETOX PROGRAM

Elimination/Hypoallergenic Dietary Guidelines

> ***Organic fruits and vegetables if possible.*** Make sure you wash them thoroughly to remove pesticides and contaminants. Be sure to read labels on all products thoroughly to find added ingredients and avoid anything with sugar, glucose, fructose, EDTA, flavoring, color, or any other preservatives.

Vegetables

Vegetables to Eat
All fresh vegetables (try to incorporate onions, garlic, carrots, beets, leeks, celery, cauliflower, Brussels sprouts, cabbage, green beans, broccoli, asparagus, leafy greens—kale, mustard greens, turnip greens, bok choy, kohlrabi etc.)
Sweet potatoes, yams
Can be eaten raw, steamed or baked, no frying.
Try sprouting, especially mung beans, alfalfa and red clover, as they help with detoxification.

Vegetables to Avoid - Corn, mushrooms, peppers, potatoes

Fruits

Fruits to Eat
All fresh fruits
Fruit sauces (applesauce, apple blackberry, apple cherry) with no added sugar (Santa Cruz or Wellesley's apple sauce)
Eat fruit by itself a half-hour before or two hours after a meal, unless using in a fruit smoothie.

Fruits to Avoid – Bananas, citrus (oranges, grapefruit), melons, strawberries, dried fruits

Grains

Grains to Eat
Brown rice, millet, buckwheat, quinoa, tapioca, teff, amaranth
You can also eat cereals made from these grains.
Brown rice pasta

Grains to Avoid - All gluten-containing grains (wheat, spelt,
    rye, oats, barley) commonly found in breads, pasta, and
    other products from refined flour
Avoiding these foods for a few weeks gives your body a chance
    to relax. You may not even know you have an allergy to
    these foods because the symptoms may be so subtle.

Legumes

Legumes to Eat
All legumes (adzuki beans, navy beans, black beans, etc.)
All peas (fresh/split/snap)
Lentils (any variety)

Legumes to Avoid - Soybeans and soy products (tofu, soy milk,
    soy sauce, miso, tempeh, TVP) as soy is another common
    allergen

Nuts and Seeds

Nuts and Seeds to Eat
Almonds, macadamia nuts, sesame seeds, Brazil nuts, hazel-
    nuts, pecans, pumpkin seeds, sunflower seeds, walnuts, all
    in their raw form

Nuts to Avoid - Peanuts, pistachios, cashews, and any nuts or
    seeds that are salted or flavored in some way

Animal Products

Animal Products to Eat
Free-range chicken and turkey (can be grain-fed if organic is not available)
Organic lamb, wild game
Wild deep-water fish (salmon, halibut, cod, mackerel, sardines)
Sparingly use eggs, butter, and cheese

Animal Products to Avoid - Red meats (beef, pork, bacon), sandwich meats, hot dogs, sausage, canned meats, smoked meats, shellfish, catfish, dairy (milk, cream, sour cream, yogurt)

Condiments

Condiments to Eat
Oils: only olive and flax oil
All herbs (e.g., parsley, coriander, garlic, ginger)
All spices (e.g., curry, fennel, cayenne, basil, cinnamon, clove)
Sea salt
Spreads: tahini paste, nut butters (e.g., almond, hazelnut, sesame, sunflower), apple butter (Eden Organic), bean dips (e.g., hummus)
Sauces: pesto, mustard with no additives
Apple cider/brown rice vinegar, fresh lemon juice (not concentrated)
Sweeteners: stevia, monk oil
Don't heat flax oil. Instead, mix into cooked grains, drizzle over salad/steamed vegetables/grains, or add to a fruit smoothie.

Condiments to Avoid - Regular table salt, refined oils, margarine, shortening. **All sweeteners** (corn/brown rice/maple syrups, molasses, honey, brown/white sugar, glucose, maltose, malt dextrose, MSG, etc.). This includes desserts and all processed foods high in sugars.

Beverages

Beverages to Drink
Filtered water, at least eight to nine glasses per day
100% fruit and vegetable juices (e.g., Ceres juice from South Africa has a variety of juices that are not sweetened)
Herbal teas: try Bija teas (nice combinations), rooibos (black tea), peppermint, chamomile, licorice root, passion flower, dandelion, milk thistle (the latter two teas are excellent liver detoxifiers, try one cup/day), and any other herbal tea
Green tea
Rice milk (Rice Dream Pacific) and nut milks (Breeze, Pacific)
Decaf coffee
Try warm water with a ¼ squeezed lemon in the water; it aids digestion and liver detoxification.
Drink liquids ½ hour before or one hour after eating, or it will dilute the enzymes in the stomach needed to properly digest the food.

Beverages to Avoid - Caffeinated beverages (coffee, black tea, soda), alcohol, dairy (milk and other dairy products), soy milk, all fruit drinks high in refined sugars, all vegetable drinks high in salt

MEAL SUGGESTIONS

Breakfast

Breakfast may include combinations of approved grains, meats and fruits. Here are a few ideas:

Porridge:

- *Buckwheat/millet/brown rice (Bob's Red Mill Creamy Rice Farina) porridge or quinoa. To this you can add cinnamon and apples or pears, a few almonds, and rice or almond milk.*
- *Add fruit, nuts and spice to porridge while it's cooking; makes fruit and nuts more digestible and adds flavor*
- *You can even mix buckwheat and millet together!*

Fruit smoothie - blend together the following:

- *1 cup rice/almond milk*
- *1 cup of fruit (berries, pears, mango)*
- *1 tbsp flax oil*
- *1/2 tbsp tahini*
- *a few almonds*

Cereal

- *Buckwheat flakes (Arrowhead Mills), rice flakes (Arrowhead Mills), rice crisps (Barbara's), nutty rice (Pacific Grain Products) cereal with rice or nut milk*

Lunch and Dinner

Lunch and dinner may include approved organic/grain-fed chicken and turkey, wild game, fish, grains, legumes, cooked or raw vegetables, soups and salads.

Snacks

- *Brown rice crackers or brown rice cakes with almond butter and sugar-free apple butter, tahini with vegetable topping (sprouts, cucumber, cooked beets), avocado*
- *Fruits, especially those that are seasonal*
- *Raw vegetables (carrot and celery sticks)*
- *Handful of nuts or a baked sweet potato*

Food Reintroduction

It will be up to you to decide how long this diet is to be continued for (usually it is recommended to follow this diet for at least three weeks, but do note that six weeks is optimum). Once the elimination diet comes to an end, you will be gradually reintroducing the foods that you have been avoiding.

Every newly introduced food or food group should be eaten during at least two of the three meals in one day for three consecutive days. At any point when you start to react to the food, you need to stop eating the offending food. If, however, you have no reactions after the third day, you simply introduce another food group.

Please note that when you react to an introduced food, wait until your reaction subsides prior to reintroduction of the next food group, and do not eat the food that you reacted to until the reintroduction of all the other food groups is over. Then, add the food group at the very end.

Here is the list of food groups that need to be reintroduced into your diet. Please note that the following order can be altered depending on your situation and what you may prefer.

- *Dairy (milk, cream, sour cream, cheese, butter, yogurt)*
- *Red meats (beef, pork, bacon)*
- *All gluten-containing grains (wheat, spelt, rye, oats, barley) commonly found in breads, pasta and other products from refined flour*
- *Corn*
- *Tomatoes, mushrooms, peppers, potatoes*
- *Eggs*

- *Caffeinated beverages (coffee, black tea, soda)*
- *Shellfish, catfish*
- *Soybeans and soy products (tofu, soy milk, soy sauce, miso, tempeh, TVP)*
- *Peanuts, pistachios, cashews*
- *Bananas*
- *Strawberries*
- *Citrus (oranges, grapefruit)*
- *Melons*
- *Dried fruits*

Once you have reintroduced all the various foods into your diet, you need to go back and try eating those foods to which you were sensitive. See how you react to them again. If you have any adverse reaction(s) to that food or food group, then you know that you may need to avoid that food/food group all together or eat it sparingly.

Some additional tips from Dr. Rasa include the following:

- *CoQ10: 100mg daily*
- *Fish oil: (EPA being at least twice the proportion to DHA): 1000 mg in total*
- *1 glass of lemon water in the morning, before anything else.*
- *1 glass of celery juice /day (1/4 can be of other fruit such as ginger, pineapple, beet, apple, etc.)*

Modifications:
Eggs are OK to eat.
Coffee can be reduced gradually and stopped within one week if needed.
Honey can be used sparingly.
No frying, no preservatives, no preservatives
No table salt – sea salt or pink salt in moderation

YOU CAN DO THIS—IT'S JUST 21 DAYS

The detox is not a diet. Eat eggs, chicken, fish, most fruits, vegetables, nuts (especially almonds, walnuts, Brazil nuts, pecans, and macadamias) in the proportions that you desire. I did cheat only in the area of adding tomatoes, a must for salads for me, plus they really do not affect you on this program. Your salad dressing of choice will be olive oil and fruit vinegar with a big squeeze of a fresh lemon or lime juice. But sprinkle some meat, chicken, fish, shrimp, cheese, and sun-dried tomatoes on your salads for variety. If you can find some dietary or almond flour bread (probably found at an organic supermarket) with no sugar on the label, a little diet toast with butter and a touch of honey will be a nice break from time to time. But be careful of honey and use it moderately, if at all. Also, you will find that homemade guacamole will be a popular addition to put on your food and snacks.

And your new best friend for the 21-day detox will be carbonated water with ice and a wedge of lime. It will be the closest thing to booze that you will taste for 21 days.

I suggest you make this detox as fun as possible. Perhaps do it with somebody else. Your challenge will be preparing the meals or finding good vegetarian, keto and vegan restaurants. Perhaps some deliver. Come up with your own recipes. I was making three to four egg omelets cooked in olive oil with jalapeño, onions, olives, tomatoes, and cilantro. Also, chicken thighs with the skin, braised and baked with veggies and a sugarless maracuja or orange sauce with spices. I ate all kinds of salads to which I added any kind of meat, chicken or fish. For salad dressing use olive oil, fruit vinegar, salt, pepper and fresh lemon/lime juice. I not only got used to it, but it is all I use now for my salads. The key is to not cheat and watch what happens. And be fore-warned that, like getting off any drug, there will be some withdrawal problems during the first week. You may feel tired, low energy, or even depressed. But by day six or seven you will see new energy, feel better, and start noticing aches and pains disappearing. Just stay with the program for only 21 days and see the difference.

Not one day was I hungry or feeling starved, yet after 21 days, I lost 22 pounds without even trying. This was not my purpose in detoxing, but it was a nice additional bonus. Now I typically will do a detox one to two times per year just to fine tune my metabolism and health, and I will typically lose three to five pounds when doing so.

If you do the detox, I would love to hear from you and your comments would be welcomed at **richholmanmedellin@gmail.com**

LET´S FREE DR. RASA FROM IRAN!

I have written *Killing You Softly* because I want to give back, save some lives, and help people improve their health. We are all in this together, and as citizens of the world, we cannot always depend upon our governments and big corporations to be truthful or to always have our backs. As discussed earlier, I would not be here today or have written this book without my original detox, which was provided by Dr. Rasa Nikanjam.

If you do the detox and it has improved your health and life (or shared it with someone who has had positive results), then consider helping Dr. Rasa.

After I met her in 2016, she got divorced from her Colombian husband, Gus, and left Colombia, moving to Costa Rica with her son. She received no financial support and was living on an organic farm just getting by and taking care of her autistic son. You can imagine how tough it is for any immigrant who is basically abandoned in a foreign country. Because of some visa issues in Costa Rica, she ended up moving back to Iran and then got locked in during the pandemic. Now she and her young son would like to leave Iran but cannot afford to do so.

In Dr. Rasa's own words from a recent email,

"Since the riots that happened in Iran last year, life has become very unsafe, especially for dual citizens, like me. Many dual citizens have gone missing, kept as hostages, or were arrested with the accusation of being spies. I have lost that connection with Latin America that I once had. But I still love the Latino culture. So, I've been thinking about perhaps Latin America, Portugal or Spain. My dream is still to set up that healing center somewhere safe in nature. Even though it's been so far from my reality for years, I'm still holding that vision alive."

I want to help Dr. Rasa, and hopefully, you, with your newfound health and personal miracle, will wish to do the same.

Accordingly, I am dedicating 10% of the profits from the sale of *Killing You Softly* to assist Dr. Rasa to relocate from Iran. I did send her some money to her Paypal account (which she set up in Canada). Her Paypal account is dr.nikanjam.nd@gmail.com. Feel free to send her a donation if you feel so inclined.

I tried to set up a GoFundMe account to assist her but I was denied because she is in Iran. I find that ironic as she wants to escape from Iran and her son is a Canadian citizen, not even Iranian. She is a dual citizen, both Canadian and Iranian. You can imagine the scrutiny she is under by the authorities there. She very much wants to leave and use any funds raised to not only live in a Latino country, but to establish her own holistic healing clinic, to save lives again, as she did mine. I hope that we can all assist her in this endeavor.

CHAPTER 21
A HEALTHY FUTURISTIC FUTURE

It is hard to imagine 20 years into the future when the Sugar Industry's days are numbered. Just like Big Tobacco, people are going to figure it out.

But what will our food consumption pattern and landscape look like?

Some of my friends, who also are my critics, tell me that we cannot exist without Big Food in its present configuration. They ask, how do we rewrite and replace our present food system?

I do not have the answers, but I have some ideas. I also will tell you what I do know for certain. People around the world are basically smart and good. If given the right tools and opportunities, people can do great things. The only things that get in their way are bad government and bad people.

In Colombia, I see such a great entrepreneurial spirit. An intelligent hustle and bustle that has overcome huge obstacles but, as a country, is on its way to greatness. I see what it is like to be an immigrant and how immigrants in any country come not just to survive but come with a sense of "fresh eyes" and fresh ideas. They do not always see the status quo.

As the world wakes up from its sugar slumber, I know it will have fresh eyes as it energetically acclimates itself to healthy eating, exercise, and sleep—and for the first time, living longer, better, and happier.

I have confidence in what an enlightened and motivated government and populace can do. In my future I see mandated healthy living that will involve novel planning and implementation along with tremendous incentives such as the following:

- 100% of doctors will receive **intensive nutritional and endocrinology training** in medical school.
- **Preventive medical clinics** will be in every town, city, and street corner.
- **SEA (Sugar Eaters Anonymous)** will replace AA as the nation's #1 support group.
- **Tax credits and monetary incentives** will be given to any citizen who starts a **garden in their front yard**, back yard, rooftop, balcony, country plot, etc.
- Every day **fleets of fruit and vegetable trucks** will pick up produce throughout the country from its citizen farmers and provide them with monetary credits or fruit and vegetable barter slips. Fresh produce will be delivered daily to supermarkets and other grocery stores and distribution centers. This way more people will be getting ripe, tasty, fresh fruits and vegetables instead of unripe produce that is ripened with ethylene gas in trucks and warehouses.
- **Healthy cooking classes** will be mandatory and taught in every grade school, high school, and university.
- All citizens will receive government credits or funding for joining gyms, bicycling clubs, swimming clubs, organized sports teams, running clubs, yoga, etc., often with medical direction and assistance.
- **New *slow* food franchises** will emerge like Keto King, Sweet & Sugarless, Energy Max, Longer Life, Macro Deluxe, Biome Blasters, McHealth's, etc. There will be special Michelin stars awarded to the most tasty and creative healthy-eating restaurants.

- Processed food will be reformulated with an emphasis on fiber, nutrients, vitamins, minerals, protein, healthy saturated fats, and sugar replacements like stevia, monk oil, and honey. In fact, this is already underway but sadly, not in the unenlightened United States. Dr. Robert Lustig and his team are already working with one of the largest processing food companies in the Middle East as apparently somebody there has read Lustig's book, *Metabolical*. They are working on redesigning the formulas to make that food more palatable and healthier. It is a beginning.
- Mothers will receive strict prenatal diet training with the **things to be avoided during pregnancy**: drugs, alcohol, smoking, processed foods, and sugar.
- Huge tax incentives will be provided to encourage more organic farming to increase production and lower prices.
- **Legislation will be passed** to break up corporate farming and bring back small independent farming that adheres to non-pesticide, natural fertilizer and non-GMO farm practices.
- All USDA **sugar and corn subsidies will be eliminated**. New subsidies will be enacted for organic farming.
- For non-organic produce farming, strict rules will be in place to be sure that fertilizers and pesticides are closely investigated and regulated to be sure there are no trace elements or chemicals that can affect public health.
- The USDA will introduce **soil revitalization programs** including remineralization of soil, use of natural composts, introduction of microorganisms, reduction of nitrogen-based fertilizers, and similar programs.
- **Vertical farming** will increase 100-fold.
- **Aquaponics** will be the norm and an integral part of society.
- With the world now eating right and exercising, good sleep will be facilitated. Sleep therapy will be part of the preventative medicine clinics and the goal will be for all citizens to get seven to eight hours of sleep each night, without pills.

- Well-constructed medical IRA programs will once again be launched that will give all citizens monetary incentives to stay healthy.
- **The number-one drink in the world will be water**, and without Coca Cola using so much of it, there will be a lot more to go around. Efficient water desalination plants will be located worldwide, not just in the Middle East. All public water supplies will be carefully monitored for any trace elements of destructive chemicals or bacteria.
- **Medical schools will have a new curriculum called Preventive Medicine**, and it will become the number-one specialty. It will not only include implementing the Big Three (eating real food, exercise, and sleep), but also proven methods that work for holistic medicine, ancient Asian medical techniques, biofeedback, anti-aging protocols, proven herbs, spices and supplements, acupuncture, chiropractic therapy, intermittent fasting, and other remedies.
- **Glucose monitors** will be provided for free to all citizens.
- The use of **antibiotics in feeding farm animals will be halted.** Corn and soy will be reduced or eliminated from their diets.
- Artificial meats will be closely regulated to be sure that the formulations are not detrimental to good health and protect the liver and feed the gut.
- **Sugar and processed foods will be treated like tobacco:** taken out of schools, hospitals and public places, taxed and with label warnings on all packaging. Age restrictions to purchase, similar to alcohol and tobacco, will be implemented. There will be public-service announcements showing how sugar fries your brain and leads to dementia. The mainstream media will do front-page news coverage about how to stay healthy and how sugar hurts health. Positive human-interest stories will abound about happy people reclaiming their health.

- AI will play a big role in this transitional period of the world reclaiming its health. I can see AI assisting in cultivation, growing, and distribution of real food. AI will have a hand in preventative medicine—perhaps at each preventative medicine center you go to an AI healthy monitoring station before checking in with a doctor. You give Dr. AI a sample of your urine, you stick your arm and hand into the machine, it pricks your finger and takes your blood pressure, does an immediate scan of your medical history, takes your temperature, looks at your eyes and mouth, examines your saliva, measures your bacteria, and prints out a diagnostic info slip that you take to the receptionist. She, he, or another AI bot will now send you to one of the preventative medicine doctors based upon your info slip information and the urgency and type of your initial diagnosis. This will all be streamlined and free.
- There will be plenty of new industries emerging to replace parts of Big Food, Big Health, and Big Pharma. So, there will be a shifting of jobs and money during this transition. We do know that supply and demand work, and this will be no exception.
- Due to life expectancy in the US continually increasing and now at 87 years of age, the government will announce that the social security benefits age of eligibility has been raised to 75 years.

This is just a short list, and some people a lot smarter than me will envision a much longer list and many more opportunities for implementing change and making money. Some other people—let's call them naysayers—will ask, "Who is going to pay for this?" and "Will people buy into this?"

For starters if 75% of the US healthcare budget is $3.2 trillion USD, that will pay for all of this. Remember that 75% of the US healthcare budget is for treating largely preventable chronic disease. That number is staggering and represents the fifth-biggest GDP in the world. Let's put it to use where it will do some good. People will buy into it once they have either experienced the miracle of a detox or when it becomes uncool to be unhealthy. People will not want to miss out on being on the healthy bandwagon.

In the United States we see that without making tobacco illegal, we have made it uncool. You cannot smoke anywhere these days except in the privacy of your own home (and there are even second-hand smoke issues arising there). Smokers are herded into small smoke-filled fog-like glass enclosures in airports to puff away or they are huddled outside restaurants or workplaces, in the cold and rain, puffing on their cigarettes with fellow smokers. The majority of non-smokers will not even date smokers. Basically, smoking is not cool anymore, and the same will happen for sugar and processed-food eaters. There will not be fat-shaming, but there will be few excuses for being overweight anymore. It will not be cool to be overweight, and there will be no need to be overweight. No more plus-size models at fashion shows. It is not that there are not healthy fat people, or that you are a bad person if you are fat, but there will be a lot more motivation not to be fat.

What will be fun to watch is the unleashing of the creative entrepreneurial spirit worldwide as we move to a future of eating real food, exercise, and sleep. I hope that I am here to witness this. The world can do this and the Sugar Industry cannot, and will not, stop us. This I know.

CHAPTER 22
FINAL WORDS

This is my very first book and it has been both a revelation and a labor of love. Perhaps when I turn 100, I will write a sequel about how getting off of sugar allowed me to enjoy my years from ages 80-100 and how during that time, I ticked a lot of items off my bucket list.

My reward for finishing *Killing You Softly* is a trip to Thailand, which will be one more item off my bucket list. Some new items for next year and my 80th birthday will be to take up yoga and body-building for seniors. I also plan to buy a small farm one to two hours from Medellin that has fruit trees, a vegetable garden, water, laying hens, and perhaps access to some fishing. Maybe I will give marriage a second chance, who knows? I do know for sure that there will be no cake or soft drinks at my 80th birthday party, but perhaps a nice glass of malbec will be in order.

We should all keep in mind that over millions of years our wonderfully developed human bodies were not designed with sugar in mind. Sugar consumption is a new phenomenon, and evolution has not had time to adapt to it. You and I will not be around, if and when that day occurs. So, you need to help Mother Nature by quitting eating the thing that is destroying your health: sugar.

I really hope that each reader will do the 21 day detox and then dedicate themselves to getting the word out about sugar and processed foods. If the ground swell is large enough, perhaps in less than 20 years we can all beat the Sugar Industry by getting the attention of our politicians. At some point they will have to act.

In closing, I wish each and every reader the utmost happiness and good health, and I hope that each of you can say what I can: that the last quarter of my life has been my best quarter.

ACKNOWLEDGMENTS

I never planned on writing a book, but after my health was restored from simply giving up sugar seven years ago, it was a combination of anger and research that created the desire to give back. My life had been saved from what I believe was a miracle, so the first person whom I wish to thank is God. My anger was stoked by my research, and the more I discovered about the corruption in our food and health care, the madder I got. I became determined to tell the truth about sugar even if it never made me a dime. If I could save just one life, then all of this effort is worth it.

Because most people did not believe I would ever write this book, my list of supporters and influences is a short one. My brother, Ed, has always been supportive, but every once in a while, I could hear him snicker as I rambled on about the perils of sugar. But I think he is beginning to be a believer, and over the past year has been sending me articles and ideas. He has even cut back on his tequila. My very dear friend, Jeff Fell, who lives in Philadelphia, has had a number of good ideas and probably believed more than anybody that I was going to complete this mission. He has tossed out several good ideas, especially in the cover design. My friend Mike Shotay has been an indirect inspiration for believing in this book as Mike is older than I am but is in even better shape than myself; he is already a strong adherent to eating real food, drinking minimal alcohol, and incorporating a vigorous exercise regimen. Finally, I would mention that seeing Dr. Tom Walsh's newfound vigor after he detoxed and got sugar out of his diet motivated me all the more to get this book finished.

I need to thank my publisher, Sierra Melcher of Red Falcon Press & Red Thread Publishing, as without meeting her I probably would have kept procrastinating about finding a publisher since that is a subject that I knew nothing about. But this was part of the miracle. My HOA was putting in a new elevator in my building; it was going to take four to five months to replace it, and I live on the tenth floor (220 steps). At age 78 I decided to look for a furnished place to rent and only looked at one place: Sierra′s apartment. While there, she said she had a publishing company. I did not rent her place, deciding to walk about 50,000 steps instead over the next 5+ months, However, I did feel it was fate that I met her on my singular rental apartment exploration and hence engaged her services. My editors, Mimi Rich and Ali Atkinson have also been helpful.

The real heroes who deserve my recognition and gratitude are the truth-telling, anti-sugar crusaders who allowed me to fact-check and verify that *Killing You Softly* is not a book of fiction. It starts with Dr. Richard Jacoby and *Sugar Crush*, which got me started on my journey. This led me to the godfather of the anti-sugar movement, Dr. Robert H. Lustig. He inspires me even to this day to want to go back and take some classes in biochemistry and endocrinology so that I could completely understand what is going on at the cellular level. Following him has left no question in my mind that sugar is deadly and reaping harm on the entire planet. Closely aligned and covered in my book is the original anti-sugar truth teller, John Yudkin, who died unrecognized, unappreciated, and forgotten. Well, not anymore—if I could only dedicate this book to one person, it would be to John Yudkin.

Some other shout-outs have to go to some of the more inspirational conveyors of truth about sugar such as Gary Taubes, one of the few non-doctor authors who brings a very strong credible research acumen to the table, castigating sugar in the process. I loved the books and podcast interviews by Dr. Richard J. Johnson, whose wry sense of humor and anthropological bent made sugar's dark side really stand out. Dr. Joel Fuhrman is very motivating in his podcasts and books and can easily make you a sugar hater as well. I personally found *Drop Acid*, by Dr. David Perlmutter, interesting as neither I nor any of my doctors ever talked about my uric acid levels being out of tolerance. Now I know why, and now they are within tolerance since I quit sugar. There are many great podcasts that cover our health, but the ones that I enjoyed most, and touched many times on sugar and fructose, were those by Dr. Peter Attia, Dr. Andrew Huberman, and Dr. Aseem Malhotra. Two other great information sources have been the Kick Summit series conducted by Florence Christophers and the Quit Sugar Summit series with Mike Collins.

These are great symposiums for those fence-sitting sugar addicts who need some additional motivation and inspiration to quit eating poison. In fact, my very first podcast was with Florence Christophers, and I will be returning again now that this book is finished. I need to mention my dentist, Juan Carlos Mejia Escalante, who has been faithfully providing the best dental care of my life and who was an early witness to my array of cavities, crowns, root canals and plaque-ridden teeth. After quitting sugar, I have been rewarded with no cavities, no more drilling, and a mysterious disappearance of plaque. Juan Carlos was the first to notice my miracle a year after quitting sugar when he asked, "What have you been doing?" And I thought, "OMG, another crown or perhaps something worse." But he said, "You do not have any plaque. What have you been doing?" I told him my story about sugar and my detox, and after that he detoxed and dropped 15 pounds; he is now a strict anti-sugar advocate, his energy is through the roof, he follows anti-aging protocols, and he has promised me he will buy a copy of my book.

Lastly and possibly most importantly, where would I be without that lovely spirit, Dr. Rasa Nikanjam? In reading *Killing You Softly* you know that she was part of the miracle by being in that interview with her husband and sharing her detox program with me, which led to my life-saving miracle. If this book has any success, and it inspires people to dedicate 21 days to Dr. Rasa's detox program to improve their health, maybe we can help Dr. Rasa and her son to depart from Iran. If we are wildly successful, perhaps there will be sufficient funds for Dr. Rasa to start her own clinic in Latin America, Spain, or Portugal.

To that big, beautiful world out there, I will simply say without good health all other priorities seem to lose importance. I sincerely hope that you try the 21-day detox, you quit eating sugar, and that you live your last 25 years better than your first 25 years.

THANK YOU

If this book has been helpful to you, we ask you to leave a review and/or share it with a friend.

It only takes a moment to leave a review on Amazon amzn.-to/47M69XN or Goodreads.com.

Thank you so Much. Your review means a lot.

ABOUT THE AUTHOR

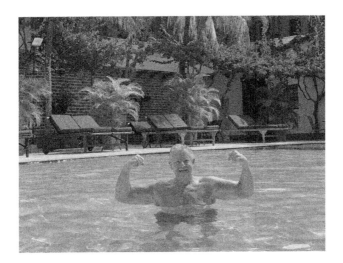

Rich Holman

Rich Holman As a result of his deteriorating health, he discovered that sugar and processed foods were the cause. He healed himself by making simple changes and now provides insights not covered by current health professionals, researchers, and the literature.

His passion is saving lives by exposing the perils of consuming sugar; he offers a free, attainable solution. Rich has had a varied U. S. business career in the real estate, mortgage banking, securities, publishing, and investment banking industries. He holds a BBA degree in Chemical Engineering Management from the Univ. of Texas and an MBA from the Ohio State Univ.

Prior to moving full time to Medellin in 2007 and starting his first real estate company, Rich lived in Naples, FL, Atlanta, Los Angeles, Minneapolis and Boston. He is originally from Texas where he resided for 12 years.

In 2007 Rich started a real estate company to assist foreigners to purchase properties in Medellin. By 2019 the company had grown 110 employees with offices in six cities and three countries. Post pandemic he launched his new real estate company, Primavera Realty Medellin.

After seven years of research, Killing You Softly is his first book, a hard-hitting expose of the world´s biggest killer – sugar. He was dying seven years ago and now at age 79 he is in great health, off of all meds and is living proof what can be achieved by doing one thing –quitting sugar.

richholmanmedellin@gmail.com

ABOUT THE PUBLISHER

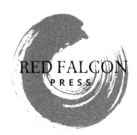

Red Falcon Press, is on a mission to publish human stories the world doesn't get yet. Our Authors share powerful stories missing from the cultural narrative. Our Readers are hungry for insight, transformation & healing & to feel seen & represented in the books they read.

A Non-fiction Imprint of Red Thread Books
www.redthreadbooks.com

Red Thread Publishing is an all-female publishing company on a mission to support 10,000 women to become successful published authors and thought leaders. Through the transformative work of writing and telling our stories we are not only changed as individuals, but we are also changing the global narrative & thus the world.

www.redthreadbooks.com

See our catalog of books:
   bit.ly/RedThreadLibrary

Our partner imprints work in parallel with our mission to empower previously silenced voices.

Vision: Changing the world for a more just, open global society. A Community of passionate, forward-thinking humans lending their genius to the collective through books.

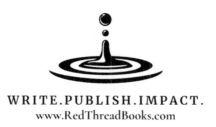

WRITE.PUBLISH.IMPACT.
www.RedThreadBooks.com

facebook.com/redthreadpublishing
instagram.com/redthreadbooks

NOTES

4. WHAT IS SUGAR?

1. LUSTIG, DR ROBERT. *Metabolical: The lure and lies of processed food, nutrition, and Modern Medicine*. S.l.: YELLOW KITE, 2021, p 14.
2. Bonner, Bill. *Insider-Outers A major change in the primary trends, from politics to finance to society at large... DEC 21.*

6. IT'S A STACKED DECK

1. "Dr. Paul Lynn, MD: Medical Doctor: San Francisco." SFPMG, January 29, 2021. https://sfpmg.com/dr-paul-lynn-medical-doctor-san-francisco/.
2. https://Www.Statista.Com/Statistics/1377721/Lobbying-Spending-on-Pharmaceuticals-and-Health-Products-in-the-Us/, n.d., Feb 2023.
3. https://Www.Opensecrets.Org/News/2023/02/despite-Record-Federal-Lobbying-Spending-the-Pharmaceutical-and-Health-Product-Industry-Lost-Their-Biggest-Legislative-Bet-in-2022/, n.d., Feb 2, 2023
4. "CDC Pressed to Acknowledge Industry Funding." *ASH Clinical News*, November 2019.
5. Judith Garber. "CDC 'Disclaimers' Hide Financial Conflicts of Interest." *Lown Institute*, November 6, 2019.
6. Staton, Tracy. "Merck Recruits Ex-CDC Chief as Vaccine Leader." *Fierce Pharma*, December 22, 2009.
7. Jewitt, Cristina. "F.D.A.'s Drug Industry Fees Fuel Concerns Over Influence." *New York Times*, September 15, 2022.
8. Piller, Charles, and Jia You. "Hidden Conflicts? Pharma Payments to FDA Advisers after Drug Approvals Spark Ethical Concerns." *Science*, July 5, 2018.
9. Foley, Katherine Ellen. "Trust Issues Deepen as yet Another FDA Commissioner Joins the Pharmaceutical Industry." *Quartz*, July 1, 2019.
10. "Five More Pharmaceutical Companies Join NIH Initiative to Speed Therapeutic Discovery." *National Institutes of Health (NIH)*, June 12, 2012.
11. McGrail, Samantha. "NIH Ties Up with Top Pharma Companies for COVID-19 Drug Discovery." *Pharma News Intelligence*, April 20, 2020.
12. Tanne, Janice Hopkins. "Royalty Payments to Staff Researchers Cause New NIH Troubles." *BMJ* 330, no. 7484 (2005). https://doi.org/10.1136/bmj.330.7484.162-a.
13. Andrzejewski, Adam. "Anthony Fauci Defended NIH Culture Of Secrecy – The $325M Third-Party Royalty Complex. Now We Know More Details." *Open The Books*, August 9, 2023.

7. HOW THE SUGAR INDUSTRY DISTORTS THE TRUTH

1. Robert H. Lustig, *The Hacking of the American Mind: The Science behind the Corporate Takeover of Our Bodies and Brains* (New York, NY: Avery, 2018), p 81-82.
2. Robert H. Lustig, *The Hacking of the American Mind: The Science behind the Corporate Takeover of Our Bodies and Brains* (New York, NY: Avery, 2018), p 277.
3. Robert H. Lustig, *Fat chance: The bitter truth about sugar*. London: Fourth Estate, 2013, p 10-11.
4. Robert H. Lustig, *The Hacking of the American Mind: The Science behind the Corporate Takeover of Our Bodies and Brains* (New York, NY: Avery, 2018), p 277.
5. Robert H. Lustig, *Fat chance: The bitter truth about sugar*. London: Fourth Estate, 2013, p 113.
6. Robert H. Lustig, *The Hacking of the American Mind: The Science behind the Corporate Takeover of Our Bodies and Brains* (New York, NY: Avery, 2018), p 275.
7. Robert H. Lustig, *Fat chance: The bitter truth about sugar*. London: Fourth Estate, 2013, p 242.
8. Robert H. Lustig, *The Hacking of the American Mind: The Science behind the Corporate Takeover of Our Bodies and Brains* (New York, NY: Avery, 2018), p 216.
9. "Big, Fat Disappointment: Dietary Guidelines Are Broken, and Government Again Failed to Fix Them." *Washington Examiner*, Editorial, July 20, 2020.
10. Robert H. Lustig, *The Hacking of the American Mind: The Science behind the Corporate Takeover of Our Bodies and Brains* (New York, NY: Avery, 2018), p 7.
11. Lustig, Robert H. *Fat chance: The bitter truth about sugar*. London: Fourth Estate, 2013, p 278.
12. Robert H. Lustig, *The Hacking of the American Mind: The Science behind the Corporate Takeover of Our Bodies and Brains* (New York, NY: Avery, 2018), p 278.
13. Robert H. Lustig, *The Hacking of the American Mind: The Science behind the Corporate Takeover of Our Bodies and Brains* (New York, NY: Avery, 2018), p 277.
14. Ruskin, Gary. "New Paper: Coca-Cola's Influence on Public Health Conferences and Groups." *U.S. Right To Know*, December 1, 2022.
15. Ruskin, Gary. "IFIC Misleads the Public about Diet, Health, Ultra-Processed Food." *U.S. Right To Know*, October 30, 2022.
16. Berens, Michhael. "How Doctors Buy Their Way out of Trouble." *Reuters*, May 24, 2023.
17. O'Connor, Anahad. "Sugar Industry Long Downplayed Potential Harms." *New York Times*, November 21, 2017.
18. Mohney, Gillian. "Sugar Industry Paid for Medical Review in 1960s That Downplayed Link Between Sugar and Heart Disease, Report Finds." Episode. *ABC News*, September 13, 2016.
19. Robert H. Lustig, *The Hacking of the American Mind: The Science behind the Corporate Takeover of Our Bodies and Brains* (New York, NY: Avery, 2018), p 94.

9. SUGAR SCIENCE FOR DUMMIES

1. LUSTIG, DR ROBERT. *Metabolical: The lure and lies of processed food, nutrition, and Modern Medicine*. S.l.: YELLOW KITE, 2021, p3.
2. Joslin Diabetes Center. "High-Fructose and High-Fat Diet Damages Liver Mitochondria Increases Fatty-Liver Disease Risk and Metabolic Syndrome." *Science Daily*,

October 1, 2019.

10. THE DISTURBING TRENDS OF SUGAR CONSUMPTION

1. Diamandis, MD, Peter H., and Raiany Romanni. "Abundance 360 Metatrend #15: Disrupting Healthcare. Dematerializing, Demonetizing & Democratizing Health." *Abundance 360 Metatrend #15*, January 27, 2023.
2. Rogers, Kristen. "Eating Too Much 'Free Sugar' Has 45 Negative Health Effects, Study Finds." *CNN Health*, April 5, 2023.
3. Brody, Jane E. "The Downside of Having a Sweet Tooth." *New York Times - Personal Health*, July 22, 2019.
4. "Noncommunicable Diseases." *World Health Organization (WHO) - Health Topics*, September 16, 2022.
5. *#194 – How fructose drives metabolic disease | Rick Johnson, M.D. Peter Attia M.D. Podcast Series*. Accessed February 7, 2022. https://peterattiamd.com/rickjohnson2/.
6. Piore, Adam. "Americans Are Addicted to 'Ultra-Processed' Foods, and It's Killing Us." *Newsweek*, December 8, 2021.
7. Goel, Akash, Michele Nischan, Bill Frist, and Tom Colicchio. "The US Food System Is Killing Americans." *CNN Journal*, August 7, 2020.
8. Tulleken, Chris van. "It's Time to End the Tyranny of Ultra-Processed Food." *Wired*, June 30, 2023.
9. Lustig, Robert H, Timothy S Harlan, Rachael V Gow, Andreas Kornstädt, and P. Wolfram Alderson. *The Metabolic Matrix: Re-engineering ultra processed foods to feed the gut, protect the liver, and support the brain*, March 30, 2023.
10. Sullivan, Kaitlin. "Metabolic Fundamentals Delivering Essential Science and Perspective on Metabolic Health." *Levels*, December 12, 2022.
11. O'Connor, Anahad. "Unhealthy Foods Aren't Just Bad For You, They May Also Be Addictive." *New York Times*, February 18, 2021.
12. Hyman, MD, Mark. "YOUNG FOREVER (PART 2): 5 STEPS TO EXTEND YOUR HEALTHSPAN." *Moonshots Mindsets - PETER H. DIAMANDIS*, April 13, 2023.
13. Bruno, Brigida A, Dorothy Choi, Kevin E Thorpe, and Catherine H Yu. "Relationship Among Diabetes Distress, Decisional Conflict, Quality of Life, and Patient Perception of Chronic Illness Care in a Cohort of Patients With Type 2 Diabetes and Other Comorbidities." *Diabetes Care*, July 7, 2019.
14. Chen, Elaine. "Diabetes Will Be 'a Defining Disease of This Century' as Global Cases Are Set to Surpass One Billion by 2050." *STAT*, June 22, 2023.
15. "Ties Between Alzheimer's Disease and Diabetes." *Brain Health Registry*, February 28, 2023.
16. Mosconi, Dr. Lisa. "The Road to Alzheimer's Disease Is Lined with Processed Foods." *Quartz*, March 23, 2018.
17. Wadyka, Sally. "The Link Between Highly Processed Foods and Brain Health." *New York Times*, May 4, 2023.
18. Dolan, Eric W. "Ultra-Processed Food Consumption Linked to Adverse Mental Health Symptoms." *Psy Post*, October 12, 2022.
19. Brenan, Megan. "Americans' Reported Mental Health at New Low; More Seek Help." *Gallup - Well Being*, December 21, 2022.
20. Kekatos, Mary, and Youri Benadjaoud. "One-Third of US Teen Girls Seriously Considered Attempting Suicide in 2021: CDC." *ABC News* , April 27, 2023.

21. Kaplan, Bonnie, and Julia J Rucklidge. "Junk Food and the Brain: How Modern Diets Lacking in Micronutrients May Contribute to Angry Rhetoric." *NeuroScience*, December 9, 2021.
22. Livingston, Bob. "Bob Livingston Alerts." *Personal Media Liberty Group*, March 10, 2018.
23. Piazza, Geri. "How Diet May Affect Age-Related Macular Degeneration." *National Institutes of Health (NIH)*, June 6, 2017.
24. Suh, Sunghwan, and Kwang-Won Kim. "Diabetes and Cancer: Is Diabetes Causally Related to Cancer?" *NIH National Library of Medicine* , June 1, 2011, 193–98.
25. Boseley, Sarah. "Sugar in Fruit Juice May Raise Risk of Cancer, Study Finds." *The Guardian*, July 10, 2019.

13. WOMEN'S LOVE AFFAIR WITH SUGAR

1. Friedrich , Cathe. "Why Women Crave Sugary Foods More than Men." *Cathe*, June 27, 2017.

16. THE TOBACCO TEMPLATE FOR SUGAR REDUCTION

1. Mclallen, Lyda. "Sugar vs Cigarettes: Which Is Worse For You?" *Diabetes Daily* , April 2, 2016.
2. Campbell, Jean. "Who Owns Your Food? Big Tobacco Execs, That's Who." *In Fitness And In Health* , January 19, 2022.
3. "Big Food: Sounds A Lot Like Big Tobacco." *Center for Science and Healthy Living*, January 1, 2022.

18. KISS (KEEP IT SIMPLE STUPID)

1. "List of Diets Wikipedia Https://En.Wikipedia.Org/Wiki/List_of_diets," n.d.
2. Carter PhD, Jen. "That Diet Probably Won't Work Long-Term — Here's What to Focus on Instead." *The Ohio State - Health and Discovery*, February 1, 2022.
3. Engber, Daniel. "Unexpected Clues Emerge About Why Diets Fail." *Scientific American*, January 13, 2020.
4. Rumsey, MS,RD, CSCS, Alissa. "The Science Behind Why Diets Don't Work." *https://alissarumsey.com/why-not-to-go-on-a-diet/*, December 3, 2021. https://doi.org/Alissa Rumsey, MS, RD, CSCS,.

19. THE ROLE OF SUGAR IN ANTI-AGING AND PREVENTIVE MEDICINE

1. Janin, Alex. "The Longevity Clinic Will See You Now—for $100,000." *Wall Street Journal Health & Wellness*, July 10, 2023.

Printed in Great Britain
by Amazon

34567750R00116